# Ways To Lose Weight
## 4 Part Series

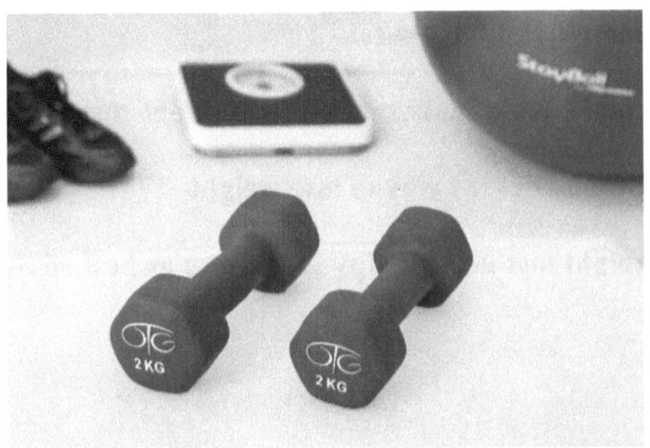

**By Jay L Miller**

# <u>Chapter 1: Introduction</u>

Do you want to have an extra great figure? Then, lose that extra weight instead!
If by chance you are now reading this e-book, then cheer-up and better gear up your loin. You are just in time for the right realization of your dream. This is the genie that will make a wish of having a wow body be made to a reality. This e-book is designed to help the reader achieve the ideal body weight by losing the extra unwanted weight in a healthy way. This e-book made a compilation on the best possible means and mode that has been proven effective for years already from different scientific breakthroughs with the most effective and safe way to lose weight focusing on the needs and aspects of a woman as a gender. The details and ways of weight loss techniques found in this e-book which has been proven for several years with different experts behind it.

As a saying goes 'experience makes a best teacher', truly the same holds true. In this e-book, different real-life experiences and testimonials are made available. The truth on the most effective ways and means to trim and extra flab and fats is being exposed in this e-book. This e-book will carefully and effectively teach you on how to cut-down on extra fats and weight at a desired pacing and timing without compromising overall and specific health state and condition of a person or a woman whose goal is to have a desirable weight and attractive fit body and physique.

As weight gain is most likely to be associated and attributed to food intake and food quality. It is not just as plain and simple as cutting down or limiting food intake as a way and solution to weight gain. Other consideration should be investigated as well.

Food is never bad. In fact, it is the ultimate fuel of the human body. Like in nay case, moderation of anything that is taken into the body would always be the basic rule. The amount or quantity as well as the quality of food taken in by the body are the considerations that would really matter most.

Binging on food would be most likely the major cause of obesity and weight gain especially amongst women. As food binging would be the most common tendency and a form of immediate self gratification most specifically in women who are so engrossed with work or career. Being so busy with a task or job would most likely cause a person to skip meals then overeat after as a form of compensation for the missed meal.

Stress and over work pre-occupation would be the major culprit and contributing factor for weight gain and obesity as one's mind gets so engrossed with work. The tendency of a person would then be to forget what goes inside the mouth and how often one goes also. Due to stress as well, a person would commonly retire to bed or throw oneself in the couch for good movie marathon with bunch of popcorn or curls as a reward for a whole tiring day. This would also be a cause for a person's inactivity and lack of physical exercise. As a consequence of such, the weight of a person increases.

Weight gain may not be sudden or abrupt to some but may also be surprisingly fast and noticeable amongst other women. This specific behavior would become a routine and habit then could later be a lifestyle to most of the career women in this case.

On the later, you would already be surprised with your vital statistics which have all one up. The once sexy coca cola bottle curve and shape has now turned to a coke in can shape. For sure, with all of these attributes not only as physical change which can be observed but most significantly a change in health status or condition would be noticed. You would now see the remarkable change in your health state and much worst you might end-up suffering from an illness or a debilitating heart complication problem out from a sedentary and unhealthy lifestyle.

***You still have time to work on those extra pounds!***

Now, as you may notice the remarkable difference in your weight and how you look and as well how you feel with your own body and health for sure would be awaken with these loud alarms. You now realize the need to lose weight and regain your health status as well. Most commonly, one would feel and experience minor health problems as an implication of sudden weight gain. Other people who suddenly gained large amount of weight would commonly complain of discomfort, uneasiness, sudden shortness of breath usually preceding an activity, feeling of depression, and the worst would be isolation of oneself coming from low self-esteem and self confidence due to altered self-image that is brought about by undesirable physical change with weight gain.

The worst thing or scenario in gaining weight would be heart complications. Heart problems would just surprise one and would often attack one offguarded. The prevailing and disturbing issues would cause ne to confide and ask the advice of a doctor or a professional health specialist. This time, the doctor or the health professional would first address weight gain problem and issue through a weight loss regimen or program.

Definitely, getting into a right diet and proper exercise would not be an easy task at all. In fact, it is even the most difficult and the most challenging part. This holds true most especially with women who are career oriented and would most often spend their time working. Time is a valuable and precious thing that a woman should battle for. This e-book will help women to decide on what diet or weight loss program to pursue that would best suit one without compromising on quality time spent with work and life and at the same time gearing to the goal of maintaining physically fitness and optimum health all at once. This e-book will help you not just by helping you obtain your most desired weight but at the same time help you live a healthy lifestyle.

***The most common reasons why one is not losing weight as intended:***

You must be annoyed and probably feel disappointed after all the effort exerted just to lose weight and still no remarkable effects are being seen and felt. Do not get impatient and give-up right away. Try to reassess and check if you are making the right steps correctly or not. Try to sort the possible things which could have contributed to such dilemma. Also, try to examine if you are just overwhelmed and may have gotten things too fast. It is important that you should really have the thorough understanding and knowledge as to where you are in your diet regimen and program. Also, know your strengths and weaknesses because in this way you will be able to improve and do something about your weaknesses. In this phase, it is also important to know if you are doing the details of the diet program or exercise correctly and as prescribes and expected from you. These specific areas for assessment and questions would lead you to the right answers and would help you decide as whether you should continue the program that you are currently engaged into.

This e-book will help you thoroughly understand the possible reasons on why things did not turn-out to be the way you expected things to be with your diet regimen. Why does it seem that all your efforts in dieting are deemed ineffective?

***You could consider the following reasons:***

- Most probably your diet program does not perfectly and rightfully suit you and your specific needs. You should bear in mind that every person has different needs. One mode of dieting may perfectly be effective to others and may not hold true to be effective with you. It may not be as what another woman would claim that's effective with them. Physical exercise is a very important element in losing weight. If you would really want to effectively burn those extra calories, then you have to get into your feet and find the right exercise program that would perfectly suit and fit you and your needs in losing weight. Also, you should make sure that you are doing it regularly as well. Cardiovascular exercise is an important form of weight loss exercise. This could help you effectively lose weight if done at least five times a week with at least 30 minutes everyday. If you are just a starter, slower your pace or until your body adjust to it.

- Another factor which also holds true would be lack of regular sleep. A daily good amount of sleep is very important in pushing through with effective diet and weight loss regimen. When a person lacks the prescribed amount of sleep, the tendency would then be that the person will resort to food binging as to compensate for the lack of sleep. This would be a normal tendency and coping mechanism of the body when deprived of the essential and basic need. The body would increase the production of the appetite hormone called or known as cortisol due to the lack of sleep. It will also be further discussed on the later portion of this e-book. Remember that you should take an 8-hour sleep every day to maintain a healthy and balanced health.

- Also playing a crucial role in one's diet and appetite would be stress and anxiety. These factors which are common are the modern-day culprit of weight gain and obesity. Taking the example, when you are stressed out or feeling anxious. Your tendency is to resort on comfort foods as these would give you immediate 'feels good effect'. By taking a chocolate bar or sundae from pantry would give you the immediate comfort. This can in turn be a form of a habit and would make you grab for more. Eating sweets and food rich in simple carbohydrates or food high in sugar would tantamount to a sudden and fast weight gain. It would most likely double your pound. It is best advised that when you are caught to be in a stressful and anxious situation, you should simply just take a moment to relax and breathe calmly. You can find in the chapter of this e-book on how to effectively deal and manage stress and anxiety.

- Overeating is also one of the major culprits in weight gain and obesity. Eating all the calories not needed by the body anymore would in turn be stored as excess fat and pounds in your body. Learning how to manage and control the amount and the quality of food taken in is very important in a weight loss or dieting program. Moderation of whatever is being taken in should be kept in mind all the time. Self-discipline would be an important consideration to control overeating.

- Eating nutritious food consistently is an issue in weight loss and dieting as well. You should remember that it is not all about the amount and quantity of food taken in the body that would make you gain weight easily. Also, a great factor would also be the quality of food taken in. though you may eat small amount of food but would grab a slice of a cake or a scoop of ice cream every after one would make dieting futile. To lose extra pound, self- discipline and being conscious of what one eats would also be important.

These are just some of the common reasons on why one does not get the desired weight or lose the desired amount of pounds given the time. If you feel guilty and feel that you have committed one or more of the stated and enumerated factors do not lose hope still. This e-book will help you understand thoroughly on how to battle and deal with the proper way of losing weight. This e-book is designed to be easily understood by common readers. There are no jargons or complicated medical terms that would make things hard to understand and complicated for you. This e-book will help you do things right the first time and all the time!

## Chapter 2: Contributing factors on why one does not lose weight

Nobody would want to be labeled as obese or fat, right? In this sense majority would want to gear and have a desirable body by all means. Any man would aspire for a chiseled chest that would make a head turn for women. And all women would want to have an eye-popping curvy figure as any man would desire. The ideal weight for a man who is standing 6 inches and one centimeter tall should be not more than one hundred eighty pounds to be exact. While a woman who stand five inches and six centimeters tall should not weigh more than one hundred and forty pounds.
Ideal and as well not easy to be maintained or attained by men and women at all. Because of this, many men and women would commonly take his to the common and known fad on dieting and losing weight. One may enroll into taebo training to eliminate extra fats and some would be engaged and join belly dancing sessions to desperately get rid of the extra belly fat.

What if none of those are working for you? This is where the dilemma comes in. With such a problem, this e-book is made from a compilation of the different effective books for effectively losing weight and proper dieting.

This e-book has cited 5 different and most common factors like the ones found earlier in this e-book which are the reasons for one who could hardly lose the excess weight and pounds. It is suggested that you have to really read and understand the details discussed and taught in this e-book.

**The following factors are:**

1. Lack of physical exercise
   - Physical exercise is the most important and essential thing that should be incorporated in one's diet regimen or weight loss program. If you would wish to shed off the extra flab and achieve a desirable body contour and shape then proper exercise is a must. You really have to sweat out the excess calorie taken into your body. Exercise would be the ultimate way to eliminated extra calorie deposited in your body. A good cardio exercise would be the most common and effective form of exercise. Pacing would vary per individual though. As earlier stated in this e-book, on should consider the pacing of a cardio exercise according to the body's condition and capacity until such that body will be able to adjust finely with the desired pacing

2. Lack of sleep
> As also previously been discussed in the earlier chapter of this e-book, the lack of a regular and complete sleep is one of the major contributing factors on why one would not effectively lose weight at all. A regular eight hour sleep every night is needed by the body. There is a tendency that the body would require more amount of food and spend less energy basing from a study with woman who sleeps less than five hours in a day.

3. Stress and anxiety
   - Stress and anxiety as one of the major factors with ineffective weight loss for women. Stress and anxiety would cause a person to binge in food as an alternative or a way to compensate such. The normal defense mechanism of the body is to eat and resort on comfort food. As the hormone cortisol is being secreted by the body to increase appetite, this would be the reason as to why one would easily get the extra weight over a short period of time. Also associated with stress and anxiety would be the lack of interest for activity. This would also be a reason for a person to gain extra weight resulting from inactivity.

4. Overeating
   - If one eats a lot, then one would gain weight as a logical reason. It is very important that one should be conscious of what goes inside and how much goes inside the mouth and subsequently into the body. A balance diet and a nutritious meal are very important. Quality of food intake should not be compromised even when under a diet program. One should be conscious and mindful that the body should still get the desired and right food when even under a diet regimen. As one would control the quantity of food taken in.

5. Inconsistency in exercising and diet
   - Eating nutritious food consistently is an issue in weight loss and dieting as well. You should remember that it is not all about the amount and quantity of food taken in the body that would make you gain weight easily. Also, a great factor would also be the quality of food taken in. though you may eat small amount of food but would grab a slice of a cake

or a scoop of ice cream every after one would make dieting futile. To lose extra pound, self- discipline and being conscious of what one eats would also be important.

These are some of the major factors and reasons why one does not get the desired weight or does not lose weight at all. It is not only important to have a fit and curvy body, but as well a much bigger importance and emphasis on a healthy lifestyle as well.

## Chapter 3: Health Issues behind weight gain

Weight gain is commonly attributed to food intake. Yes, it is a fact that food can be the most common reason for weight to shoot up. But, is not the ultimate truth in all cases. The reason and a consideration why one would have a sudden increase in weight despite of the tremendous effort being exerted on dieting and exercise.

This would be attributed to some underlying health conditions or diseases. There are common health conditions and diseases which are believed to be the reason and culprit of the unceasingly obvious weight gain.

The following are the most common health conditions:

1. hypothyroidism
2. food sensitivity
3. Cushing's syndrome
4. post partum
5. organ disease
6. prescription drug use
7. anxiety
8. blood sugar imbalance
9. essential fatty acid deficiency

Let us discuss each of the following stated health condition for a thorough understanding and knowledge of these:

1. hypothyroidism
   - ➢ Hypothyroidism is an underlying factor in weight gain wherein the bodies insufficiently produce the hormone thyroid by the thyroid gland.
   - ➢ Thyroid hormone regulates the metabolism in both animals and humans. A deficiency of such hormone in the body would result to slowing down of body's metabolism. Though a loss in appetite is being experienced by a person, but ironic to it would still be the significant increase in body weight. Weight gain is brought about by fat deposits associated with fluid retention caused by protein deposits in the body that would in return increase weight of a person.

➤ The most common signs and symptoms experienced by a person with hypothyroidism are the ff:
a.  fatigue
b.  lethargy or sleepiness
c.  swelling of the face or around the eyes
d.  dry skin
e.  course skin
f.  decreased sweating
g.  poor memory
h.  slow speech
i.  hoarse voice
j.  weakness
k.  headache
l.  intolerance to cold

2.  Food sensitivity

The most common notion and perception for food sensitivity would be allergic reactions following specific food intake. Food allergies do not just cause one to feel itchy and see remarkable physical allergic appearance. One of the effects that food sensitivity would cause would be weight gain. The effect of the allergen taken into the body may not be immediate. The reaction to which may take several minutes or even hours. An overt symptom would right away follow as manifested by swelling and bulging of the body. Weight gain may be observed right after the allergic attack.

The following are the signs and symptoms being experienced from food sensitivity:
a.  headache
b.  indigestion fatigue
c.  depression
d.  joint pain
e.  canker sore
f.  chronic respiratory symptom
g.  heartburn

3.  Prescription Drugs

Research has shown that people who use prescription medicines everyday gain large amount of weight. Furthermore, research proved that prescription drugs increase the appetite of a person. In this case, possibility of weight gain is really to be considered.
Another prescription drugs which can cause weight gain and increase in appetite would be oral contraceptives in women. Oral contraceptives would cause fluid to be retained in the body, thus bloating and increase in weight can be observed.

4.  Essential Fatty Acid Deficiency

Deficiency in fatty acids in the body would trigger one to crave for fatty foods. Since, the human body needs essential fatty acids for metabolic functions, insufficiency of which will cause the body to compensate. The most common signs and symptoms of a person with essential fatty acids deficiency would be the following:

a.   dandruff
b.   dry hair
c.   dry and scaly skin
d.   mouth ulcers
e.   increased susceptibility to infection
f.   poor wound healing

Essential Fatty Acid Deficiency may be associated as well with the following health conditions:

a.   arthritis
b.   eczema
c.   heart disease
d.   diabetes
e.   premenstrual syndrome


5.  Cushing's syndrome

Cortisol is an important hormone in the body that is being produced by the adrenal glands. Cushing's syndrome is developed due to an overproduction of cortisol a hormone in the adrenal gland. This known health condition causes weight gain to a person very quickly. Fluid retention in the tissues of the body causes this substantial weight gain of a person. People who are suffering from this kind of condition would have the definite characteristic of a 'moon shaped face'.

The following are the definitive signs and symptoms found in the person with Cushing's syndrome:
a.   buffalo hump on the neck or shoulders
b.   arms and legs are often not proportion
c.   spots on the face chest or shoulder
d.   headaches
e.   back pain
f.   skin darkening on the neck
g.   skin becomes thinner and easily bruised
h.   bruises and scratches as well as insect bites take time to heal
i.   reddish-purple stretch marks found in the abdomen, buttocks, arms, legs or breast
j.   in women, menstrual period becomes irregular
k.   frequent urination
l.   feeling of thirst
m.  poor libido or lack of sexual appetite

n.  some psychological problems

In this case, a person who has Cushing's syndrome should consult a professional doctor and ask for a collaborative support and treatment.


## <u>Chapter 4: How to lose weight in 1 week</u>

This e-book will really help women attain a desirable weight in a sure and doable way. As having a great figure would be any woman's desire. A slim and fit figure coupled with great abs would really be head- turning for men. Men would go crazy to see women clad in their seductive and attractive fit figure.

True enough in our society today, media and press would make loud on the issue of physical fitness and healthy lifestyle as a need and a form of compulsion. Having and working out on this quality would be an edge of a woman in life.

In this chapter of the e-book, loosing weight can be easily understood and workable even in just a week! Specific methods will be discussed. It would then be up for the reader if one would consistently do it or not. Thus, the sustainable outcome and effect will also depend on which. But before one gets into action, one of the greatest considerations would be planning. This time you should grab your calendar and star plotting on the specific dates as to when to start with the practice. See the details of how to lose weight in 1-week steps:

> **SUNDAY**

> ***<u>Face that camera, say cheese and shed pounds</u>!***


Sunday is probably the day that you usually take off, perhaps going to churches, treating yourself to a shopping spree or perhaps dining out with your loved ones (if you are on the process of working out to get that great figure you need to watch out for your diet though) or perhaps going to the nearest park to relax. You need not to change this routine, go on with it and enjoy, after all this is your day off from work. Now as soon as you come home though, the first thing that you should do is to get that camera of yours and take a shot of yourself before gobbling up your dinner and another picture as soon as you are done with your meal.
You must be wondering as to what the purpose of picture taking is? Well according to a certain study by Robert A. Carels, Ph.D., an associate professor in the psychology department at Bowling Green State University recording meals may help you lose up to 5 percent of your weight. Now those pictures that you have taken can help you with your food diary. It can help you determine the actual amount of food and the type of food that you eat. It is also strongly suggested that you download the pictures you have taken so you will have a record of it.


- **MONDAY**

> ***<u>Take that multivitamin</u>***

Monday, you might probably be in a rush, taking that early morning shower and gobbling all that calorie full breakfast. Why not? You must be in a work for hurry, trying to beat that traffic jam unless you leave 10 steps away from your workplace. But wait before you get to absorb in your daily routine just to get yourself to your workplace, what about your diet? Your goal is to get that perfect slim body! Do not forget it nor take it for granted. Now to beat this Monday rush, here is what you need to do according to two studies in the British Journal of Nutrition they suggest that taking a daily multivitamin may make you less hungry and those people who take multivitamin tend to weigh less and have lower body mass index (BMIs).

So start your day right, pop that multivitamins which have 100% recommended daily allowance (RDA) of vitamin and mineral intake. Take note that these vitamins and minerals chromium, copper, folic acid, iodine, manganese, molybdenum, niacin, pantothenic acid, riboflavin, thiamin, vitamins B6 and B12, and zinc should be in your multivitamin to support the need of your body.

- **TUESDAY**

> ***Burn those calories by speeding up!***

Tuesday might be a little hectic than Mondays. You have gotten yourself back on track. Now add this to your calendar. Try to wake up a little earlier than you used to do, say an hour before your usual waking up time. Now here is what you need to do on this Tuesday morning. According to Jim Stoppani, Ph.D., author of "Encyclopedia of Muscle and Strength," strength-training circuit-style burns more calories than the traditional way. Apart from great calorie burner strength-training circuit is also perfect for travelers or for people who want to get more done in a short period of time. Now bear in mind that in circuit training the shorter the rest period between sets, the more calories you blast off. So what you need to do today is to start that circuit exercise by doing one set of 15 reps for each exercise with no rest in between; wait 20 seconds and repeat the circuit twice.

- **WEDNESDAY**

> ***Torch more fat by taking triple dose of that Big C!***

Vitamin C has multi functions. Ascorbic acid is not just use to boost your immune system or to shield any skin allergies that you have, Vitamin C is also used to lose weight. According to research in the Journal of the American College of Nutrition, if you regularly consume 500 milligrams or more of vitamin C it can help you burn 30 percent more fat while working out. So starting today, treat your body with Vitamin C enriched food like citrus fruits, broccoli, and cantaloupe.

- **THURSDAY**

> ### *Grab a friend and get into exercise session to drop weight*

Having a friend to do work out sessions with you will not just help you lose weight faster but you won't be able to notice the time that pass you by while you are doing exercises. Also if you have weight loss network will help you get motivated in working out to speed up your slimming goal. It is easy to turn to someone whom you know just in case you are encountering some difficulties.

- **FRIDAY**

> ### *Colors can also make you slim!*

True enough, varieties of colorful fruit and vegetable can help you maintain a great figure or can help you speed up your slimming process. For sure you have heard of the old saying that goes like this "an apple a day will keep the doctor away" and so does pounds. An easy way to cut your calorie load is to fill up your diet with a range of fruits and vegetables. Your best bet is to follow the rainbow diet. Cereals will be best if they're added with blue berry, snack on apples, and load your lunchtime salad with carrots, tomatoes, and peppers.

- **SATURDAY**

> ### *Inhale it and fight your cravings!*

Ever had the feeling of gobbling food whenever you are feeling stressed out? Most of the times, when you feel anxious or stressed out, your hunger shoot up as well. It is best to practice the yogic breathing to offset this. When you are relaxed, you do not experience much hunger pains as compared to when you are worried. Add the fact that when you are stressed out you tend to cherry pick sweet food. The loads of ice cream and chocolates increase when you are anxious. You can make rational choices on your food intake if you are relaxed. You can also do the 12-minute workout where you have to rest your right thumb near your right nostril, ring finger and pinky by your left nostril. Then you have to close the left side and inhale through the right for four counts, finally close your right nostril and hold for four counts and open your left nostril and exhale through that side for four counts. Do the same cycle on the other side and continue alternating for about a minute and soon you will forget that cookie craving of yours.
Now you have completed your weekly calendar, make sure that you stick with your plan and practice it religiously and in no time, you will attain that great figure that you have yearn to get. This calendar of ours can be used as your guide if you are starting to take weight loss seriously. You can use this as the start of your weight loss efforts, and this can complement the other

weight loss suggestions that you can get from this eBook. We are just starting, and on the next chapter, we list the most common diets that you can note in the market.

## Chapter 5: High Sugar in diet makes weight loss efforts Futile

When you get into the thing of dieting and you are dead serious to get rid of those extra pounds, you must be certainly sure as well that you have to put a little sacrifice on other gratifying food. Sugar is the culprit of weight gain amongst the different types of foods. One should have a high sense of discipline in one's self in turning down to sweets and rich in sugar food. One should be aware of the food intake and the types and kinds of food being ingested in the mouth. As these foods would have a direct effect on your body. Most especially for those women in diet and weight loss program, awareness on the food taken in everyday is very important. It is not only significant that one should only be conscious of the quantity of food taken in but as well the quality. One should learn the different major food items, food contents, composition and be aware of its immediate effects the pros and cons of each individual food.

Sugar or high sugar in food does not only cause a person to gain weight quickly and easily but the fact that high sugar in one's diet can also pose health threats to a person. It is also the culprit in diabetic attacks. Different health ailments and conditions are directly linked and caused by high sugar or rich in sugar diet. Being aware and mindful of the details of the food which one eats will not only help the person lose weight but as well prevent pending debilitating health conditions.

The following are the foods which are high and rich in sugar content that would be detrimental in ones health and as well makes dieting and weight loss efforts futile.

> **White flour**

- One should be conscious of food made of white flour.

- White flour will make your blood sugar rise as much as what the refined sugar can do. And when you get too much of the white flour, then your intestines are the ones that will definitely suffer. There will be intestinal infections that can be attributed to the consumption of white flour.

- White flour is hard to chew. Too much pressure on the digestive system and this is low on fiber.

- The following are the examples of food items that may contribute to your weight that are made from white flour will include:

    a. bread

    b. cakes and pastries

    c. Pastas

Moderation is the key if you really want to eat food items like these. It is also important to note that any food items that are made from flour have no nutritional value at all and these things may only cause more harm than good to your body so be aware of these things.

➢ **Carbonated drinks**

- It is a known fact that soda and carbonated drinks do more bad things than good, and these drinks also deliver the extra pounds for the person.

- A can of your favorite soda will contain 15 teaspoon of sugar, 150 empty calories, caffeine plus the drink is also loaded with lots of artificial colors and flavoring. You need to be aware of the fact that drinks of this kind is dangerous too since this may contain artificial sweeteners.

➢ **French fries and donuts**

- These forms of food can add extra pounds as well.

- French fries and donuts are now known and classified as junk foods.

- These food items are nice and very delicious to eat but remember that these can be your enemy when you are planning to slim down.

- French fries and the donuts are deep-fried starches. Before these food items are fried, these are your simple sugars. And the moment these are fried, then their nutritional value is then lowered once again.

- You also need to remember that all fried foods will contain a number of things that may do harm for your body and your health.

➢ **Commercial energy bars**

- Commercial energy bars can also help you gain extra weight.

- Replacement bars are getting the attention now since most people are looking for quick energy and quick fix, and these commercial energy bars deliver what people want.

- These energy bars can give you that quick energy boost, but in terms of nutritional value these energy bars don't really deliver on their promise.

- Almost all of these energy bars have high sugar content. At times you can find energy bars that may contain some nutrients, but this is rare.

➢ **High sugar cereals**

- You can also gain extra pounds on high sugar cereals. Though cereals are basically known to be beneficial and can be a good source of nutrition due to its high fiber content. But having high sugar on which would convert its benefit to a disadvantage.

- For this reason, you need to consume these food items sparingly.

- Some of the more popular breakfast cereals are often packed with the simple sugars that can give you that much needed boost, but in the long run this can give you more health troubles than good.

➢ **Cookies and candies**

- These are foods which cause for weight gain. These products are often full of sugar. These products may contain sugar at high levels.

➢ **Ice cream and desserts**

- Ice cream and desserts can also add up the extra pounds on your weight. These foods are also indulged in sugar and starch which can quickly make you gain extra pounds. These foods should be eaten sparingly.

The foods or types of food mentioned above are definitely some of the most common foods which should be eaten sparingly and as much as possible to be avoided most especially by women on diet or weight loss regimen. These are the food items that are rich in sugar and as such you need to stay away from these food items. If you stay away from these food items, then your slimming efforts can go on smoothly. You will no longer need to exert too much effort or you need to revert to medications just to get the results that you want. By knowing these things and by avoiding these food items, then you can say that your weight loss efforts can go on with less issues and less hurdles. Not only one would get and have an effective diet regimen but as well would live a healthy lifestyle.

## Chapter 6: South Beach Diet the way to lose weight

In this modern era where everyone is conscious of there physique and health, people would resort by all means just to have a fit body and a healthy lifestyle. In talking about gender and to compare dieting and being conscious as to the weight and shape, women would be much on the edge on this. Women also are the ones who gain weight easily and quickly due to many considerations and factors as well. With this reality, diet comes to mind.

There are many modes and known diet programs anywhere and everywhere in the world. Much more with this, each would also claim that theirs would be much more effective and effects are sustainable and lifetime in an aspect.

In this e-book, we will be talking about a known mode of dieting most especially with women. South Beach Diet will be discussed thoroughly here. South Beach Diet is a famous diet plan that is designed by cardiologist Arthur Agatston and dietician Marie Almon. This diet was designed to act as an alternative to other popular diet programs out in the market.

The initial purpose of the diet program is to prevent heart disease, but its appeal has transcended that and right now this diet is considered as one of the most popular and one of the most effective. The system and the idea of this type of diet are simple. In the simplest sense, this diet will replace the bad carbohydrates and the bad fats with the good carbohydrates and the good fats.

For women who want to slim down with the use of this diet program, then it should be noted that they should be of the age 20 or up. The diet program is divided into three phases and each of these phases will progressively become liberal. The phase one of the diet programs will last for two weeks of the diet program.

South Beach Diet is characterized by three phases:

## First Phase:

- On this phase, sugars, processed carbohydrates and fruits are taken out of the system.
- The purpose of this stage of the diet program is to eliminate the hunger cycle and this can deliver weight loss in the person.

## Second Phase:

- The second phase of the diet program will continue as long as the person wants to lose weight.
- In this stage, fruits and vegetables are now reintroduced into the diet.

## Third Phase:

- The third phase of the diet program is called as the maintenance phase.
- This now will last for life. If one would say that this diet program can adopt and can last for life, then this should be taken seriously.


This kind of diet will call for time and attention. One of the good things about this diet is that you will be given the chance to dine out and at the same time eat well. And you can make it happen by following some simple rules and you need to stick by the principles of the diet program. It really would not matter if you are a busy career woman who lacks spare time for diet. This type of diet program would make dieting attainable and doable even for busy and career women.

But, in order for a diet program to be working and effective then one should need to know the importance of compliance and obedience to the certain and specific ground rules of this diet program in order for one to really see the effect of which.

The following are the specific ground rules to consider when one is on a South Beach Diet Program:

- When dining out with friends in best restaurants then you need to consider the unprocessed, the unrefined carbohydrates like your whole grains, the whole fruits and fresh leafy vegetables. These are the things that you should select in order to stay and toe the line of the diet program.

- In dining out then you should also focus on lots of lean protein like the protein from chicken, fish and some cuts of meat. You should also prioritize the low-fat dairy and the reduced-fat cheese.

- One should carefully select the food items that are rich in good fats. Foods rich in good fats would be fishes, avocados and nuts. Also make sure that the dishes that you will eat are prepared with the use of the healthy oils like your olive oil or canola oil.

- Definitely, you should say no to the food items that are high in saturated fat like the fatty cuts of bacon and beef. If possible, you also need to stay away from processed meats like your salami.

- Make sure that you eat food items that are rich in fiber. Fiber can be sourced from your fruits, vegetables and nuts. Other food items that are rich in fiber include white bread, cakes and white rice.

- It is also important to avoid added sugar. Cola drinks should be avoided. Also be aware of the hidden sugars that you can find in dressings and the food sauces.

If dining-out can not be avoided and if it comes occasionally then just be mindful of the following strategies on how to effectively battle on high sugar and high fat temptation. Here would be some of the list of the best strategies that you can use when you are dining and eating out. Here are some of the wise suggestions:

- Have a protein snack before a date.

When you do this, then at least your appetite can be tempered, and you will no pig out on the food items that will be served in your favorite restaurants. You can eat a hard-boiled egg or you can have a piece of cheese right before your leave your home. At least by doing this, you will not be tempted to order and eat a lot when you are out.

- Set aside the breadbasket, the chips and all that stuff.

These food choices that you normally order in the past all contain ingredients that body will not like. These will contain bad and unrefined carbohydrates. And if you eat food items like these, then these can give you that immediate boost yet in the long run will only allow you to become hungrier. If this is already served in your table, as much as possible try to ignore this basket since this will not do your slimming efforts well.

- Ordering soup can be a good thing.

It is wise to order a cup of soup the moment you are seated in your table. Now consume this soup right before you take your meal. If you are planning to get your soup, consider the soup that is rich in vegetables and make sure that the soup that you will get is not cream based. Or what you can do is to order just the clear broth. The nice thing about the soup that you will order is that this will fill your tummy up and as such your hunger will be tempered and you will not be tempted to eat that much the moment the food is served in your table. And the nice thing in ordering and consuming your soup is that this will send that message to your brain that you are eating, and you will feel full soon. And since it takes roughly 20 minutes for the message to travel by the time the meal arrives then you are already satisfied, and the craving is now gone.

- In case there would be a need to order for extra, then it would be best if you can ask for extra veggies instead of starches.

In many cases when you dine out, the main course will often come with starchy side dishes for example you will be given mashed potatoes. Remember that food items like these one are not good for you if you are under the South Beach Diet. If you are going to ask for something extra, then it is suggested that you get vegetables instead. You can go for string beans or broccoli and consider these as healthy extras on your plate.

- Consider dishes that are cooked the healthier way.

Look for healthier cooking methods and prioritize these as these can help you lose those extra pounds. And along this line, it is always a recommended move if you can get away from the food items that come battered and fried. And if the food items do come with the rich butter sauce then just ask for these on the site. Consider the healthier cooking options. For example, you can go for roasted, broiled and grilled food items. Cooking options like these offer less fats and will not introduce fats that will not help you in your weight loss efforts.

- Consider alcoholic drink as not part of the plan.

But if you cannot really help it, then it is suggested that you just have a drink or two. If the waiter asks for something to drink, then better stick with a glass of water or you can go for diet soda.  You can also go for a glass of wine- red or white wine if you really want a taste of good life.

- Don't scrimp on the dessert please.

You can also go for dessert. All diets will also call for some amount of dessert. Life would be pretty boring without dessert. So, don't deprive yourself- add some fun to your weight loss efforts.

Remember these ground rules related to the South Beach Diet. Once you are aware of these ground rules, then it will be easier for you to follow the diet program and it will be easier for you slim down and cut down those extra pounds.

Commonly a fact that regular eating and dining out can add up on extra pounds. It is most true when you are not paying attention to what you are eating then this cannot help you in your weight loss efforts. So if you are one of those women who wants to slim down and to lose some weight yet loves eating and dining out, then it is important that you are guided with some of the best strategies and techniques when you go out and dine in your favorite restaurants.

## Chapter 7: Some weight loss Healthy Tips & Exercise as best advised

Now that you know some of the weight loss efforts and suggestions, it's that stage wherein you also need to realize that you need some form of exercise. Exercise is an important component to any weight loss efforts. And when you happen to check all the other leading dieting and weight loss programs out there, you will note a single thread that will govern all these weight loss efforts. All of these programs and weight loss efforts will always include a complete exercise regimen. Exercise will definitely help in your efforts to lose weight and to maintain the desired weight.

<u>Suggested exercise for weight loss</u>

- Cardio exercises
    - ❖ These exercises will deliver the goods, but the bad news is that most women tend to do it the wrong way. Remember that when you do this too much, then you risk different forms of injuries. Another mistake is doing the exercises at low intensity and finally some women tend to neglect the other parts of the programs. Other skips the strength training and flexibility just to focus on the cardio. The important key here is to balance the exercise program.
- Strength training
    - ❖ You don't need to be afraid of the heavy weights. This kind of training can also help women who want to lose weight and maintain weight.
    - ❖ Strength training is not only suited for men but for women as well.
    - ❖ This kind of training or exercise would help the body tone each muscle parts of the body, thus creating a good shape and contour of the body.

One just have to remember that no matter how good the suggestions and the tips are on how one can lose those extra pounds, if these are not backed by exercise then efforts will be futile. Exercise would perfectly complement any diet program. Living a good healthy habit is not just what one should do. The importance of a regular exercise is vital to life.

# Part 2

# Dieting - Success Guaranteed

**Table of Contents**

## Introduction

In western countries, dieting is a fad and is now becoming a daily routine for everyone. What is in dieting that everyone is falling for? Most people are more conscious of losing weight nowadays. In the study done by Mintel, one in four adults are said to be active in practicing diet and in losing weight in the United Kingdom alone. Mintel is a London based research firm which started the study of diet trends in United Kingdom. The study reveals that about 13 million people in the United Kingdom are trying on different popular diets. These findings are enough to say that dieting or losing weight is now one of the most important activities people in this country are busy about. There must be something in dieting that attracts million of followers in this generation.

Furthermore, the study shows that 37 percent of women are on at least a specific diet compared to only about 18 percent in men. That is about two in five women and only one in six for men. This is now a trend to most western countries including the United States where dieters are mostly women. For most people who do dieting, looking good is the main goal so watching out for the weight is a must. They are motivated mainly because dieting makes you lose weight and you eventually look good. The study added that people now put health and wellness a top priority and they associate it to how they will look pleasant.

This also so true in the United States where people are finding different ways to look slimmer and to look good. They are also motivated to lose weight, to look beautiful and be appreciated. This becomes the main goal for most Americans. Being healthy for them is the secondary reason and everything follows. They try different methods of dieting like low-fat diet, high protein diet or low-carbohydrate diet. It now depends on whether they want to be leaner or just slimmer. They go and find out different food choices in the market.

That is why different products and slimmer formulas are coming out to feed the need of dieters to look good. Some do not really help at all although other food recommendations are quite effective. Some people also go for natural diet which compromises mostly of fruits and vegetables rather than chemical diet or even surgery.

## Why Do People Diet

There are so many reasons why people go on diet. They have different answers depending on what they believe motivates them. You can ask your friends or your colleagues if they are on a specific diet. Most of them may have started on diet long ago or have just started. Then you can ask why they go through this process. Chances are, you will hear a lot of reasons and unique ways to have successful dieting.

For most people who have been dieting, one major reason is to look better. Probably, they want to look good because it is being required by their job. Some actors and actresses are paid to act on screen, and they are required to look their best. Models on runways are expected to be thinner.

Getting thinner; however, is difficult and poses a challenge to some because it involves changing the lifestyle and food habits. Some people go through with difficult ways and means to get thin. Some people also go for healthy options like exercise and eat more vegetables to achieve better built. For others, they just want to satisfy themselves and they experience fulfillment when they get the weight they want.

## Facts about Dieting and Food Choices

Other people have misconceptions about diet. Some think that it can be unhealthy and has bad effects to a person's general wellness. Let us square away some information about diet. Diet can be healthy when proper utilization of food and body requirements are met. For example, eating fewer calories than the normal daily body requirement poses threat to your health.

You may not notice any difference on your weight on the initial week of dieting but eventually, as the day pass, you will find that effects of dieting can be visible and can be felt. However, some people choose to eliminate the total fat from food they eat. One should remember that a little fat in food is alright but eliminating total content of fat is bad.

Our body needs a certain amount of fat that when metabolized is being utilized by the body to be used as energy. Exactly about 30 % of fat in the diet is required by the body to use as energy. It is still considered as an important part of the diet and it is recommended that no one should eat a completely non-fat diet.

## What Diet Really Means

We understand how diet has been helpful for many of us and we hear a lot of stories of diet, whether it is successful or a failure. There are different types of diet and technique available. Before we go into details about diet and how it leads to successful results, we should completely understand what diet really means. It is a now popular term and sometimes broad but we will simplify the definition of diet so it can be used efficiently and effectively. Defining diet will also help us identify what types of diet is suited for every individual.

The definition of dieting from books to online researches is somewhat almost the same. It is a process of utilizing and consuming food in regulation and is planned to meet specific requirements of individual including or excluding foods. Whether a person wants to lose weight or gain weight, dieting is a way to control a desired weight without compromising health.

There are a lot of stories about dieting from many people who already tried such process. It is a completely different story for some people in sports who maintain a well-organized way of eating and exercising to fit the needs of sports they are in. Nowadays, there are a lot available products or books about dieting. A lot of people might be overwhelmed with a lot of choices available about dieting in the market. Specific programs or types of diet are designed to meet the requirement of each individual.

There are a lot of dieting programs and trends available, but they can be categorized into only three. These are the low-fat diet, the low-carbohydrate diet, the low calorie.

1.  **Low fat diet** is a diet that is generally low in fat and is intended to help lower cholesterol in the blood. Since our body needs some good types of fats, this diet cannot completely be without fat. In this type of diet, the fat that is regulated refers to saturated fats which are mainly found in meats, lard and dairy products. These fats are also known as "Trans Fats". Limiting these kinds of fats is helpful in losing weight and in lowering the level of cholesterol in the blood.

    On the other hand, there are also "good fats" that our body needs. These fats mainly come from vegetables, nuts and fruits. They are called the unsaturated fats which are divided into three groups: polyunsaturated fats, monounsaturated fats, and omega three fatty acids. These fats are less likely to increase cholesterol level and might even help prevent heart diseases. Understanding the kinds of fat you want to regulate is important since your objective is to be a healthier person.

2.  **Low carbohydrate** diet is the type of diet that limits the intake of carbohydrate such as bread, beans, milk, rice, potatoes, and pastas. This diet is known to reduce blood cholesterol.

    However, since carbohydrates are also essential to a person's health, it is recommended that you choose the best carbohydrate foods to eat and limit those that are less beneficial. Whole grains are best options. This diet really means choosing good carbohydrates, not "no carbohydrates."

3. **Low calorie diet** is a diet that focuses on the calorie intake of the person. It limits the foods that contain most of the calories. Calories are not bad your health. These are needed by the body for energy. However, if you eat too much of it and are not burning enough of them through certain activity, you might end up gaining weight.


## How to Really Lose Weight

We have encountered a lot of different ways to get the weight we want and to have the body we want to achieve. In some instances, people would tend to follow the current trend of dieting. For example, when south beach diet booms in 2000, many people have followed the diet plan and eventually this diet has become popular to other countries. Some individuals also try to follow the diet plan of their favorite celebrities. When they see that these actors have successfully lost weight or have become more attractive after a certain diet, fans tend to follow and they become motivated to complete the diet plan.

There are still several options on why people get motivated to go on diet. For some, joining weight loss groups are effective. These groups are also effective in keeping the individuals motivated and have good percentage of completing the program successfully. There are also people who choose to make daily diaries to be able to monitor their daily food intake and also to be able to monitor their weight. This type of a diet plan is known to be effective since the food is monitored and the person becomes conscious of what he or she eats on the next meal. The person who choose to do this type of diet is readily aware of what should and not to eat and be able to monitor the calorie intake that has already been consumed.

There are also known ways of effective diet. One is through the use of medications. This is mostly popular to those individuals who are up for easy and fast. The popularity of this kind of dieting is increasing as the sales of diet medications are evident. Many people believe that these medications really work.

Though these medications are expensive, they are still patronized because they cut the time for losing weight and people do not have to stay on gyms or to starve themselves to lose weight.

Some drugs are, however being regulated for public's protection. Some medications are still in the market though they have already been prohibited. It is recommended not to use the drugs not approved by FDA so to prevent the dangerous effects even though manufacturers usually would say that their products are safe and effective. It is not really worth the risk.

Also, one of the most popular ways of losing weight is the use of water. Sometimes our body triggers sensation when we are hungry or thirsty. Very often than not, when we experience dehydration, we interpret it as being hungry and a person would eventually eat when he is actually thirsty. Drinking more water prevents overeating since you may feel full when you drink water. Always observe your body when you are hungry and when you are actually just craving for fluid.

**Questions and Frustrations on Diet**

You may know some people who have started diet. It may be your friend or your neighbor who are usually not making the effort of dieting. Or you maybe know some people who have continued to eat the foods you avoid and have not ever gone to gym but still maintain their weight and would still look better. Some people are having a hard time avoiding foods they want to eat or had stopped eating unhealthy foods but still are not losing weight. This fact frustrates a lot of people.

They ask themselves how the world has become so unfair to them. Other people though, are enjoying the benefits of not having to do the effort of losing weight and not having to go through starving or exercise. Have you ever have come to this point when you have to ask yourself why? If you arc the person who usually sticks to the diet plan or has vigorously stayed in the gym for long hours and has no better results, do not totally blame yourself. And you are not alone. There are many people who have come to this frustration. You are not alone I tell you.

Here are some of the frustrations of some who have experienced failure to dieting.

*"I started planning to lose weight when I was 26 years old. I had colleagues at work who have nice bodies and they really carry themselves well. I was envy about the fact that we eat similarly the same foods everyday and yet my weight has not changed. I even started on a low calorie diet but I failed to lose my weight. I became more frustrated when I knew that my colleagues who have beautiful bodies are not even on a diet."*

**Brad, New York**

*"Every time I look at the mirror, I get disappointed since I have done a lot of means just to lose weight. I cannot even buy the clothes I like and I cannot eat the foods I really love eating. What is more frustrating is that I don't even see my friends do the same diet I go through and they still enjoy the food everyday but still maintain the weight they have."*

**Karine, Florida**

*"I heard about the south beach my friends have tried and they got better results. When it was my time to do the plan, I did not see the results right away and when I saw the results, it was even not as better as what my friends have accomplished. I was so frustrated that I switch to a different diet I thought is much better than south beach. I ended up having the same frustration."*

**Genetically Designed versus Effort**

We would ask ourselves why it is easy for a lot of people to maintain their desired weight and still be able to enjoy the foods others are avoiding. Some people just do not make any effort. Unfortunately, for some people, it is not as simple as licking an ice cream and nothing happens. Some people have to struggle and that is always a question we want to find answers for.

There are valid reasons for this scenario. Some people inherit what they call good genes. These people have faster metabolism compared to others. Even though they would eat a lot, their bodies can still metabolize foods they take in and maintain their weight. That is partly true.

However, some researches show that metabolism is not the only reason for differences in metabolism of food. Study reveals only 50% of obesity is to be blamed with heredity. The remaining number lies on our habits. This means something important.

It means that for most of us who were not gifted by good genes can actually do it as long as we have this determination. It also means that we need to change the way we view life and the way we go about it. We must change our ways of eating, our lifestyle and must have a control over our weight. Sometimes, we are frustrated because we cannot stick to our original plans and we break the rule in the middle of what we already have started.

I am going to admit that I am one of people who also have struggled to get fit, who have tried all different kinds of methods to get the weight I have longed and dreamed of. I am going to share the long journey and the secrets I have kept. I can still say that you should continue to eat the foods you love and still be able to maintain your weight. I will tell you in details why you should eat these foods to achieve the body you want.

But before we proceed to the program, I want to share with you a bit of what happened to me before. I started on a diet a few years back. I challenge myself to make an effort of losing weight. My friends gave me a specific plan of dieting and I followed them. It took weeks and more weeks of not eating my favorite food. I usually love pizza and spaghetti. But during those times, I avoided those foods and I stick to my diet plan. You can just imagine the struggle I went through to be able to achieve my desired weight. I even have to stop eating my favorite fried chicken. I continued to pursue my program thinking it would make me look better and would give me more confidence.

It gave me results that I want in exchange to those long months of avoiding or sacrificing what I love to eat most. Was it really worth the time? Did I really enjoy the process of getting the desired weight? Did I sacrifice more than what I got?

**Secrets to Diet Success**

It was about a month and a half and it is this kind of diet plan I was into. I started to give myself a try to more of vegetables and fruits and putting a leash to my urge for delicious, unhealthy choices of food. It was the right time to really lose weight since I was to attend the wedding of my friend after two months. I would check every now and then how I was going and checked my weight from time to time. During those weeks of struggle, I began to notice that my weight was not dropping.

I told my friends that I certainly focused to my diet plan and I prepared well to those weeks when I have to change my lifestyle. I should have seen a difference in my weight as far as sticking to the plan is concerned. But why did I fail? Why was my weight the same as when I started? What was wrong with my diet plan? Is it ineffective or was it something I did?

I continued on to my program without the foods I love and eating more of the foods I never wanted to eat. Thereafter, my friend suggested that I go on a cardiovascular exercise. This was the time when I really at the peak of my struggle. I was nearly going to quit. My self-esteem was on its all time low. My weight was still stagnant. I went ahead and attended the weeding of my friend. My weight was just the same as I was planning to lose two months before this wedding day.

I realized I was standing near a table where all the delicious foods were laid. I was confident I will not participate in the food binging part of the occasion. But my friend insisted that I should go and sit with him and should have a plate of the foods they have prepared.

I decided for a long time to eat the usual foods I eat. I got spaghetti on my plate, added a piece of meat, a steak, and salads. I really enjoyed that very moment. It was an awesome feeling to enjoy what you do. I did not even think of the consequences it would bring.

The next day, it was same feeling of guilt like how other people would feel when they fail. I was pitiful and ashamed of myself since I did not accomplish the goal I originally was trying to achieve. This frustration is somewhat familiar to anyone who was trying to do the same I did and failed.

This is a very common scenario of repetitive actions of dieters. I know that some people had experienced this kind of situation I went through. Who would be disappointed of not being able to achieve the desired results when you thought you have done everything there is to do?

These results, of course have some effects on your confidence and your mentality. If you are a person who has these experiences, remember that you are not alone. After at least a week of depression, I was ready to get back on track. I tried the diet plan once again thinking that it may have a different result this time. My friend who came over from another town wanted me to join him to have fun.

He brought me some chicken that looked so delicious. So, I started to taste every bit of it and found out that I was eating everything my friend had brought me. And I was not able to stop myself.

I know that you would understand the feeling of disappointment as I went through with this event. This however did not stop me of continuing my diet. I got back to my abstinence from those delicious foods and continued my cardiovascular exercise. This time, I was not expecting better results anymore since I broke my program and I was ready to face another fact that my weight, if not the same, would go up.

When the time came for me to weigh my body once again, I was not really looking at the scale since I already had some expectations with the result. At first, I did not look closely but when I noticed a different number, I put my eyes straight to the weighing scale.

Then I saw that it was really a different number showing. I knew that I made some deviations with my original diet scheme and I knew that it was not really so enough. At my surprise, I managed to lose weight. I lost at least 6 pounds. I looked again and it seemed correct. I stood there asking myself what had just happened. I even checked the size of my waistline to confirm my result. It validated the result.

There should be an explanation to this scenario. What was going on? I knew there was something that was quite not right and I had to find out. I think you are for the revelation. What happened to me was actually out of my control. When this situation happened to you before, it was not your fault.

Some people explained that when you started regulating the food that enters your body or when you start limiting yourself of calories, the body responds to fight back the possible weight loss. It means that your mind programs your body to counter the starvation. A person who is in the middle of a crisis and has nothing to eat for a day or two does not die. The body tends to fight starvation by allowing the enzymes to be in regulation so that a person will not die. The fat burning enzymes slows down in production that is why you do not really lose weight when you starve yourself.

This is really one of the secrets of successful dieting. You will see and understand more of this concept when we go further.

The secret is to convince yourself that you are actually not on a diet so your body will not activate the emergency mode to decrease burning fat enzymes. When you achieve this type of diet plan, you will eventually get the results. You can actually eat the foods you have deprived yourselves with and still lose weight. You need to do the trick and practice this always to get better results. As you practice, you can control your weight from time to time without even putting pressure to yourself.

Read further as you are about to get the details of these secrets we are revealing little by little. Strategies will be presented so you can easily follow. The last thing we do is give suggestions that do not actually work at all. Below are the simple strategies on how to live on the secrets that are revealed.

One must understand the idea that our body triggers the regulation of fat burning enzymes a week after you made a restriction of your calorie intake. It is important that you know our bodies work so we can incorporate our steps better. It would mean that you need to plan on when to overfeed yourself and when you can cheat on diet.

These two should go together and you can also use your favorite rich foods to make this plan effective. When you start doing this strategic plan, it would change your whole life dramatically. You can assure yourself that your efforts will really pay off in the end.

When you start this unique plan, you can now forget the following situations you have experienced before:

- You do not have to be really anxious now since you know when and how to control your cravings and appetite
- You will also experience a more positive motivation and less pressure as you free to eat the foods you love while you lose your weight. You can be excited to see the results as it is effective and still can enjoy dieting without feeling discouraged.

The strategy we have presented and the secrets to losing weight are specially formulated so the person can solve issues with weight and health as well as looking good. It is time for you to have a more optimistic way of managing your weight so be assured that you will eventually have the results as soon as you have grasped its unique strategy.

You were maybe just a bystander who observes beautiful people pass by but when you start this unique plan, you can now be one of them. You can walk the streets with confidence, and you attract bystanders. Some people already have started these secrets to successful dieting, and I receive positive responses. The following are emails from one of my clients:

*I worked in an industry of models and beauties. I see them every day and they have their own stories of having beautiful bodies. Their usual way of losing weight is starving, and at least not enjoying the food they eat. They will get shocked when I told them that I still enjoy my own Rich foods and still maintain my weight. Fortunately, I do not have to struggle on my way to being beautiful*

Brian Bourne

Brian said that he was educated by the facts he learned online. He learned that our body has specific needs that we need to fully understand. He concluded that this is the only program which gave him freedom and a lot of options when it comes to choosing foods and enjoying them at the same time without feeling the pressure of gaining weight.

If you are ready to look better and enjoy life, this one is for you. It is indeed a diet of fun and freedom. We may consider if you have second thoughts or if you may not be so convinced as of yet. We understand that people today are skeptical about the products.

I received an email a few weeks back from a client who was so skeptical at first:

*I cannot believe what I just heard. Is this true? They say that this diet gives you more freedom when it comes to food choices at the same time not having to worry about gaining weight, and even lose weight. At first, I was so hesitant to try on this program since it is a completely different from the diet I usually do so it took me a week to really decide on whether I give it a try. Since my friends have decided to follow the program, I followed them and tried it since it will not harm me anyway. I started on putting my favorite rich foods on my plate without hesitation. Lastly, I ask myself if it would really work and if it is really worth the try.*

Katie, CA

Katie did not fail when she started this program. She answered her question. She has proven to herself that she can really lose weight better than before with eating her choice of foods and did not even feel the pressure of doing it. She was very happy about the results and she even told her other friends to try this unique program.

This strategy has real success stories of good results compared to other diet plans that promises beautiful, but you end up gaining more weight and do the diet all of again. You have to say goodbye to the old-fashioned way of losing weight if you want to have better results and enjoy life at the same time. The results for other diet programs are even unfortunate. Some had bad muscle tone, loose skin, they looked unhealthy and even decreased self-esteem is evident. Some diet plans do not really work at all. They are just fads.

**Comparing our Program to Traditional Ways:**

Here are the lists of comparisons that might be helpful for everyone to better understand how this program works:

- While traditional methods show that metabolism is damaged because of reduction of calorie intake, this new strategy even sustains the normal process of metabolism thus preventing abnormal reactions of body processes.


- Since metabolism is affected in old way of dieting, the moment you resume normal eating process, your original weight goes back. In the new program, when you lose the fat, it does not come back since the metabolism is protected and functions continuously in its normal pattern.

- In the new approach, muscle tissues are kept and only the fats are eradicated while in traditional ways, muscles are broken down while you are on the process of dieting since there is decreased in metabolic rate.

- In the new approach, you are always free to enjoy the foods you love without compromising your weight while old diet plan, you feel the pressure of avoiding those foods and you do not really enjoy the process. It also takes months before you see the progress of you work.

- In the old diet plan, you stick to the food choices required and breaking to the plan means that you gain weight, while in the new strategy, your intake of food is not actually measured so no pressure. You still the freedom you always wanted.

- The old approach of diet will not give you consistent results since you are always measuring the food you eat. In the new diet plan, you learn to enjoy the process and give you consistent and better results. You get the chance to see the changes in your weight every week. You do not get discouraged on the way as you continue to lose weight while having the opportunity to eat the foods you love.

- You can really attest that the old ways of dieting give you frustrations you get miserable as the days go by. You even look restless and prone to fatigue while on the new approach, you get leaner, happier and you see results. You will love the diet everyday as you go on and get more excitement when you see the results.

- You all know the kind of descriptive and labels you can attach to your old-fashioned weight loss schemes. You can always say that these dieting schemes and fads are all frustrating and miserable. But here in this new form of dieting, of course you can say that these are exciting and enjoyable. In fact, you will love every day you spent on this dieting program.

- In the old dieting programs, you will surely notice that that natural hormone levels are always down, and you know what this means right? The sex drive is down, and you feel mostly lethargic. But of course, this is not the case with this new way of losing weight. In this new way to lose weight, the natural hormone level is maintained and as such there will be an increased energy and libido.

- And finally, most of the traditional dieting programs that are available online works against the body, while this new dieting program that we have here works with your body.

So, are you going to choose the old fashion way of dieting or the new strategy we presented? I know you would choose the best option. You would choose the diet that has a lot more freedom for food and gives you more fun and excitement. You have seen the results of the new strategy and what it can do for you. It is all up to you what to choose and to discern the option that you think is beneficial to you and your body. You can either go through with the same story old dieting promises or find something wonderful in the new strategy.

Again, there are a lot of good reasons why the old strategy has failed to give better results. We have researched on calorie measurement and how it really helps us understand better the way to manage the weight of a person. We again say that these fads have continually disappointed you in many ways and now we are giving you directions on shifting to better results.

We will also have to emphasize that may not need to eat your favorite foods the whole time during the diet plan. There must be a part of the diet plan wherein we also limit your caloric intake to stimulate fat loss. It is not always eating all the way. So, we need to be proportionate with the food we take and the food we limit to make it work for us.

A lot of benefits are found on this diet plan. You are given a lot of food options in the duration of the diet from protein to carbohydrates and vegetables and fruits. It gives you the opportunity to eat the food choices you like and get the better weight you desire. You get to eat your pizza supreme or you beef steak and spaghetti. You can still eat your different sandwiches on the table. You also can consume different meat preparations and schedule the time for caloric limitations. What about your potato fries? Or maybe your fried chicken and burger, yes you can still eat them. You need to eat strategically for us to make sure that we still can get fat loss better.

So how does it work? Research says that the secret for better control of weight is manipulation of calorie intake in the body. If you can do so, you increase the chance of proper metabolism and prevent your body to starve. This plan promises you of the best way to improve weight. This new approach if followed properly can help your body acquire an effective metabolism that gives way to proper utilization of food and proper utilization of energy. You can achieve this by varying the list of food you consume every day. Your menu should include different types of food to make it balanced.

**Ways on Unlocking the Secrets**

What is in it for you and me? Here are some tips you may want to take note of:

- This e-book will provide you with the raw information about fat and the will explain why fat consumption is also essential to lose weight faster.

- You will also realize that the absence of carbohydrates in your diet is not good after all. This compilation will guide on how to use fat in proper metabolism and how they go hand in hand with carbohydrates consumption.

- You will then identify the many ways to vary your choices of in order to be of good use to really losing weight. As a result, you will increase your metabolism in order to lose weight faster but eat more.

- In this e-book, you will how to manage your meals and your time to consume food.

- You eventually will how to use the strategies in losing weight faster while enjoying physical activities available. You would be able to synchronize your diet and your activities. That gives a double time for weight loss.

You can start processing your thoughts as early as now on how to use this e-book. This will give you satisfaction you deserve.

When you decide on trying out this method we have presented, we can assure you that you will enjoy all the processes on losing weight and continually have fun. You can now start competing to your colleagues on staying slim and beautiful without having to feel guilty and pressure. You never know, he or she had been working on this unique diet all this time. He might not have wanted to share it to you since he considers this as his secret. But since you already knew this, why not start on your own get the body you dreamed of. Here are some tips on getting the best body.

- Do not think of this as a diet. If you can remember, you gained back what you have lost in your previous diet plan. When you started to regulate the food, you eat or restrict it, you gain the pounds you already lost. That was the process of the old diet, so do not follow its ways. It is always still a proportion of eating and fat loss.

- You can keep away from white bread. Studies shows that white bread are usually linked to obesity. You may want to keep away from those food choices. You may notice some people who are fond of eating white bread are usually overweight. Researchers are still on the process of identifying why this happens and getting valid evidence. While experts are not yet sure, you can keep away from it as there is no harm avoiding this food.

- You should need to trust your brain this time. Following your stomach may not be necessary. It is also common that we feel hungry and feed our stomach when we actually do not need to eat. You may to adjust your body patterns ass to identify whether your body is really hungry or not.

A lot of successful dieters do not mind eating when they feel hungry. Sometimes we associate thirst and hunger. You can just drink water. Or it sounds like it is a temporary desire of your body to taste or eat food but you are actually not hungry. You can take a walk or do something else to divert your attention to temporary desire of food.

In many cases, it goes away without you noticing it. So, when your true hunger comes, your body responds properly and that is the right time to feed your body.

- You may also consider weighing yourself daily as this would guide you in monitoring where you are at. This motivates you to continue getting better results.

- Sleeping is one important factor to consider in healthy results. Lack of sleep disturbs proper food metabolism and would eventually affect the way you control your weight. Getting enough sleep can easily help you making decisions.

- Drink plenty of water. Again, sometimes we associate hunger and thirst. You might just be thirsty and can be satisfied by drinking water. Water has no calories. You can never get wrong with it. Consider whether you are really hunger or just thirsty.

- While we enjoy our foods and we can eat them anytime, we should also consider eating fruits and vegetables as part of cleansing diet. It gives you fiber that sweeps away toxins and harmful elements in your body. Aside from that, you prevent certain diseases in the future.

- Slow down when you eat. Your metabolism determines when are full so when you eat fast, you ingest food fast and eat more and more before your body says you are already full.

- You may also want to avoid salty foods and starchy snacks as well as food high and rich in sugar. Eating these kinds of foods make you want to eat more and drink more. So it disrupts proper metabolism.


- You may also want to binge some donuts or a piece of cake at the start or at the end of the day. Enjoy those opportunities of eating such luxuries. Successful people do not feel guilty of eating desserts and these foods as part of their leisure.

You can eat these foods in moderation but not completely eradicate them.

You reward yourself with some of the best choices of food and you get the best results at the same time.

- Understand and know yourself better. Make sure you take good care of yourself. Do not deprive yourself of some special events in life when you have to eat at least more than what you usually eat. Enjoy the pleasure of undergoing a diet regimen. Be more positive and do not feel guilty.

- Before you start on any weight loss program or diet plan, measure where you started so you can identify the progress the along the way. Being able to see improvements in body shape, as well as weight, can be a useful extra boost if weight loss slows.

- In most cases, losing weight is largely a mental or emotional issue. Most dieters know what to eat and what to avoid in when eating. They know they need to take physical exercise. It's the emotional side of dieting they have difficulty with. Know what you really want and know what you need. If you want to lose weight and keep it off forever, be realistic in your weight loss goals. Don't waste time setting yourself unrealistic weight reduction targets, because you are guaranteed to fail and feel worse.

- Beware of fad diets and weight loss drugs. If you have already spent failures in previous diets plan you encountered, do not make it worse but believing that drugs would help you have faster weight loss. Stick to your plan and think positive.

- Again, we should remember that food is our friend. It gives us energy, keeps us healthy and makes us happy. We should just have to know how to use them and proper planning and consuming it.

- When you visualize being slim, you get the clear view of how you look. It is easier to lose weight when you the visualization of how you will look when you get the results. Your mind is powerful. Do not underestimate it. It is always how you think. When you think positively, you get positive results at the same time.

- The last thing you should remember is to understand your weight. It does not mean eating less. It means choosing food and choosing the right time to eat food. Do not be in a hurry. Some people fail because they rush into things and they end up quitting.

**How Exercise Helps**

Although we emphasized here on this e-book that we can achieve losing weight without to do with exercise, we wanted to also inform of the benefits of exercise and how it can help in our way to diet success. Although, exercise does not directly give significant effect on us right away, it still boosts better mood and better general wellness. When you have better mood, weight loss becomes easy. Exercise should go hand in hand with enough sleep. To be able to achieve better effects on weights loss, you may consider sleeping and exercise as part of your plan.

Here are more reasons why exercise is essential.

- It promotes better sleep. When you sleep better, you do not confuse yourself with hunger and fatigue. You may have better judgment when you get good sleep.

- o It slightly raises your metabolism. You know how important proper metabolism of food is. You may consider starting to exercise.

- o Exercise boosts motivation. When you stay active, your mind becomes active and you are happier. When you have a positive thinking, you are less likely to lose motivation.

Regular physical exercise is considered as an important part of losing and maintaining weight. It prevents several known diseases such as heart problems and cholesterol. It brings your condition to an optimum level of wellness. In at least 30 minutes of physical can really boost your health and you maintain the weight you desired. Whether you are at home, doing little chores is alright. When you walk the street, you are already doing a physical activity. You do not have to overdo it. Keeping just enough motion is already a big help to your body.

Optimism during the stage of dieting is as important as the details it requires you to do. It is somewhat a driver for you to be able to maintain the energy to continue. That is why, this compilation puts emphasis on having fun and enjoying what you do or what you eat. You always get positive results when you think positive. Just imagine if you think negative about this diet, you will eventually fail, though it is already assumed that you get the results you desired. What you think, your body follows, and you have to be careful in thinking negative as it reflects to how you do your work. Get into the habits of eating delicious food and dieting becomes easier.

## Conclusion

We always wanted to look good and to feel good. When we go up and become an adult, we get more conscious on how we look like. We try different types of dieting methods. We follow fads and trends here and there. We compete with our friends and colleagues and even to ourselves just to get the right body we wanted. We see everything on TV, we hear the news about the how people lose weight and we encounter these products to lose weights. Most of them do not really work. While everyone still struggles on the process of dieting, this e-book has already given the basic secrets to successful dieting. Some people may already have started but for those are still on the verge of deciding whether to try it out, be confident that you will get better results. It is recommended that you not only eat good food but you enjoy them at the same time. We also emphasize that you should learn the habit of eating delicious food as it becomes easier to lose weight.

Weight control methods can be successful if weight loss is maintained without compromising overall health. When you get successful in weight reduction program, you also promote permanent life-style changes. The physical and psychological benefits of maintaining the right weight can be observed when it is done are the right way. It is, however, more beneficial when you personalize the weight reduction plan based on individual's needs and lifestyle.

When you get the right ingredients of dieting like exercise and sleep, you tend to get the weight you desire. We know that getting the right weight also prevents us from certain diseases. Not only that, we function well in our daily workload. We become successful when we do our job right.

For all of us, it is definitely important that we look good. By getting the proper nutrition and understanding how the body works, we get the optimum level of health and it gives you the glow you deserve. Sometimes, we just overlooked at the secrets of getting the best of us. We miss to identify how we get through with getting healthy and looking good. Therefore, being conscious about our weight and our physical appearance is not bad at all. It actually reflects on how we live our lives and how we become effective creatures. Being healthy gives you an overall functionality.

# Part 3

# LOSE WEIGHT FASTING

Table of contents

# Introduction

The idea of fasting is still tied to the spiritual and religious practices. When we first heard about fasting, we immediately relate the term to the Catholics who practice this during Lent or to Muslims during Ramadan. In ancient times when people fasted, they believed that doing so would improve their clarity of thought and bring spiritual enlightenment and inspiration. In fact many people who fast relay a feeling of being more removed from the physical and a more spiritually focused consciousness. It should be reflected however, that having strong values is integral to this - as mental attitude is huge part of one's sense of the world.

Most would consider fasting as a spiritual enlightenment. But what is really behind fasting that those who practice it have an aura of well contentment and happiness. Those who practice them don't seem to have the effect of the environment on their physical outlook.

A few of us have tried fasting but not everyone understands its concept and benefits therefore the more we need to know on the subject to fully grasp its benefits.

For those who already are in fasting, you're further given the insights of fasting. The benefits to be fully enjoyed, one must accompany it with healthy lifestyle and healthy eating habits. Fasting is useless if we don't have the two to accompany it with the two.

As you read on, you will find a lot of information on the topic. And you near the end of this, you can be assured that you will learn more than what you expect. Then perhaps see that change you always wanted.

Take note however that results will vary with each person as each and every one of us response differently. Two people can be subjected to the same conditions and their reactions can be quite different. So never compare your results with another, what is important is that you feel that positive change in your body, mind and soul.

*"In my opinion, the greatest discovery by modern man is the power to rejuvenate himself physically, mentally, and spiritually with Rational Fasting."* ***The Miracle of Fasting*** *by Paul Bragg, ND, PhD*

# Our body

The body is a physical structure of a living thing. It is made up of cells, tissues, organs and systems that work hand in hand. They form a complex system of relationship that the absence of one greatly cripples the entire body. The loss of an eye makes it hard for our other systems to grasp the events happening around and must rely to the remaining senses.

Our body is one wonderful machine, a wonder of science. The complexity of it and how it is able to perform so many things at a time often leads it to being called the "wonder machine". It never runs out of battery, it could do work all by itself, it could even process different applications, it could come up with solutions and so much more.

Our body could do so many things that almost each single one of us are testing and pushing our bodies to the limit. We defy the laws set by nature about caring for our body. And when our body seems to be slowing down, we simply revive it with caffeine repeatedly even to the point of overloading ourselves with it.

We are in touch with our body that we know what it's capable of and sad to say, this knowledge led to the abuse of our body through the years. We eat like there is no tomorrows because we perfectly know that the body will simply digest, absorb and excrete what we eat. We drink and smoke because we know that our body has its defense system working round the clock. We drink medicines anytime we want because we know that our body could take them.

Yet do we also know that too much abuse of what our body can do is also bad? Our body is just like any machine that once it reaches its limit, it breaks down. Too much alcohol, unhealthy food and lifestyle combined with stress is extremely harmful to our body. As we age, the maximum capacity of our body will only reach its peak once and will decrease over time. Because of the decrease, our body becomes prone to different ailments and sickness, we become weak over time and if we don't heed to the pleas of our aging body, this just might cause us our lives.

It must be remembered that our body should be handled with care just as we do with other things. We must always love and care for it.


**Stress and the human body**

What is stress? It is said that stress is a condition that almost everyone can relate in an everyday sense. Stress is not new, and we are no stranger to stress. Almost everything and everywhere there is stress, there is stress in the workplace, at home at school and even in emotional perspective. And we must remember that stress will never give our bodies good benefits, in short stress never serve us well.

How a person reacts to stress differs. Stress is caused by different factors and with different resolutions. Our personality and emotions will determine how much the effect of stress on our body will be. Some may have higher stress threshold as compared to us. These people are able to meet up with deadlines calmly and still give positive results.

But the physical effects of stress on our body can be very damaging our emotional and physical health. While the effects are subtle, the long-term effects of stress are deadly. Even more alarming is the long-term effect of stress on our body. It very much acceptable to accept the fact that stress shortens our lives. Increased risk of heart disease, nervous breakdowns, stomach ulcers, tension headaches, and an increased susceptibility to infection are just a few of the things that stress can do to us. No single effect of stress is beneficial to us.

Although stress in the short run can have positive effects such as the ability to react to the situation quickly and resolve it as immediately as possible, it is never good in the long run. But, almost each and every one of us lives each single day with stress and sometimes in the succeeding years.

Stress affects our health, body and mind to such great extent that we are crippled by its effects over time. Some of the signs of stress include short-temper, anxiety, impatience, low morale, temperature changes, blood pressure increase, and migraines and so on. Yet there are times when the stress is not so hard and that person has a higher threshold, the stress condition may actually be of beneficial results that will end short with a complete relaxation.

Most often that not, insomnia and depression are the most common effects of stress on us. Because of the two, our mental and physical state is affected. Likewise, our diet is affected too which leads to our low energy levels and thus making us unproductive.

**Common ailments of the body**

As living things, we too are prone to different diseases. Despite the fact that our immune system works 24/7, it cannot battle the all the diseases that invade our system all at once. Often times the common ailments are signs of even bigger catastrophe. Not giving due attention to the common ailments will lead to something even more dangerous and deadly. A simple cold if not treated or given attention, might progress to something worse. A cough if lingers for days or weeks could mean the patient is having lung problems.

So, what are common ailments? Common ailments are simply diseases which we are prone to suffer in our everyday life. The term arises from the fact that they are occurring commonly to almost all individuals. Most common are headaches, stomach aches, pimples, acne and the list goes on.

These common ailments can be very irritating, if not disturbing for small children as they keep on coming back. This holds true for adults too. The general health of the person determines the frequency of the ailments. A person with good health and excellent immune system will most likely not be bothered with common ailments as compared to someone who isn't.

Do not be paranoid of your common ailment not unless it's worse than the usual one. These are not so serious and will be gone after a few days. A week of care and rest is usually enough for them ailments to leave the body. Do not immediately drink medicines on the first day. Try to observe fro other signs and symptoms. Taking medicine too early will mask these symptoms which could've helped in diagnosing as to the nature and cause.

There are a variety of common ailments from which people suffer from. These ailments are not very serious and can be cured by referring to some home remedies or over the counter medicines. If your ailments persist then you should immediately consult a doctor or physician.

The Common Ailments list is quite big some of them are as follows:

- Allergies
- Headache
- Heartburn
- Nasal Congestion
- Cough and Cold
- Fever/Flu
- Stomach Disorders
- Tummy aches
- Migraine
- Acidity
- Constipation

They could even be prevented. Doctors, nurses and mothers alike would all agree to the tips to prevent common ailments.

- If you are prone to cough and cold, then try to avoid sitting in A. C. for long and avoid cold drinks and ice creams as much as possible.
- If you have frequent congestion problem, then try not to breathe the polluted air outside and use a mask while going outdoor.
- Keeping yourself away from the junk food will lessen the occurrence of stomach disorders largely.
- Maintaining a balanced diet comprising, seeds, green leafy vegetables, legumes, cereals fresh fruits, and other foods enriched in vitamins and protein will help to keep the body healthy and strong enough to fight various diseases.
- Maintain the basic hygiene and keep yourself clean. Take frequent baths and wash the face, hands, and legs whenever you are back from outdoors. This will prevent development of germs in your body.
- Whenever sneezing or coughing, cover the face with a hanky.
- Maintain a proper sleeping itinerary of at least 6-7 hours and avoid stress and tension. This will help in preventing headache and other such elements. There are other significant information on the common ailments and the ways to combat it.

**Unhealthy lifestyle**

It is often emphasize that a healthy lifestyle is always the ideal one especially today that we cannot afford to be sick as the bills are very expensive. But it has been observed that our health is degenerated and we are exposed to a lot of toxins and chemicals anywhere we go. There are toxins and chemical and we are exposed every day at work, home, in the air, and in the food that we eat and water we drink.

With the fast paced life, we depend on processed food and fast foods. We have bombarded ourselves with medicines and drugs and with less exercise.

So what makes a lifestyle unhealthy? Some of the factors which make our lifestyle unhealthy are as follows:

- **Too much junk food** being put into our hands especially in children's hands. Junk food which contains saturated fat increases blood cholesterol levels and therefore increases your risk of heart disease and some cancers.

- Life is full of stress. Modern life is full of hassles, deadlines, frustrations, and demands. Work can be a stressful place, whether in an office, a factory, or a school. For many people, stress is so commonplace that it has become a way of life.

- **We are generally dependent on medical drugs** and are not aware that medical drug side effects are dangerous to their health. In the world today, many people seem to think that they just want medicines and drugs to solve their health problems; they believe they can always seek medical assistance. But what they are not aware of is that these pharmaceutical medications may have potential adverse reactions. Some drugs which are toxic to your liver and do crazy things to your health and metabolism, perhaps you obediently swallow those little poisons without considering what they are doing to your body.

- **Exposure to pollution and toxic wastes such poisonous agents from the household items**. Our bodies are absorbing the harmful chemicals surrounding the environment today. It is thus imperative that we clean up our living environment as much as possible. Those regular detergents, soaps, shampoos, toothpastes and perfumes that we uses today contain many chemicals which are toxic to our bodies, some even carcinogenic.

- **Lack of exercise**. Exercise always improves our fitness level. No questions asked bout this.

**Here enters, fasting**

Fasting often described by many books and experts as primarily the act of willingly abstaining from some or all food, drink, or both, for a period of time. A fast may be total or partial concerning that from which one fasts and may be prolonged or intermittent as to the period of fasting. Fasting practices may preclude sexual activity as well as food, in addition to refraining from eating certain types or groups of foods; for example, one might refrain from eating meat. A complete fast in its traditional definition is abstinence of all food and liquids.

Over a period of time, we all know that in the absence of food makes us weak and will have detrimental effect on our body. In fasting however, this is not always the case. Water or any fluids is consumed at quantities that satisfy thirst and other during the absence of food, the body will systematically cleanse itself of everything except vital tissue. Starvation will occur only when the body is forced to use vital tissue to survive. Although protein is being used by the body during the fast, a person fasting even 40 days on water will not suffer a deficiency of protein, vitamins, minerals or fatty acids. In the breakdown of unhealthy cells, all essential substances are used and conserved in a most extraordinary manner. There is an unwarranted fear of fasting that strength diminishes from the catabolism of proteins from muscle fibers. Even during long fasts, the number of muscle fibres remains the same. Although the healthy cells may be reduced in size and strength for a time, they remain perfectly sound.

A. J. Carlson, Professor of Physiology, University of Chicago, states that a healthy, well-nourished man can live from 50 to 75 days without food, provided he is not exposed to harsh elements or emotional stress. Human fat is valued at 3,500 calories per pound. Each extra pound of fat will supply enough calories for one day of hard physical labor. Ten pounds of fat are equal to 35,000 calories! Most of us have sufficient reserves, capable of sustaining us for many weeks.

However, fasting also has its downside. Some people do excessive fasting out of intense fear of becoming overweight. Pairing this fear with mental disturbance is very dangerous and deadly as in the cases of people with anorexia nervosa.

It must be remembered that the fasting that will be discussed in this book is for the good health and wellbeing of the individual. Never use fasting as a resort to losing weight drastically. Good results come with time.

**Fasting and its applications**

This chapter will discuss and present some applications of fasting in the fields of medicine and politics.

- Medical application. I remembered once when a family member was to undergo surgery. Her surgeon told her to fast at least 8 hours prior to surgery. If one is not familiar why the surgeon asked his patient to fast, then know that fasting is often indicated prior to surgery or other procedures that require anaesthetics. With the presence of food in a person's system, it can cause complications during anaesthesia; thus the strong suggestion of the medical personnel that their patients fast for several hours (or overnight) before the procedure. Additionally, certain medical tests, such as cholesterol testing (lipid panel) or certain blood glucose measurements require fasting for several hours so that a baseline can be established. In the case of cholesterol, the failure to fast for a full 12 hours (including vitamins) will guarantee an elevated triglyceride measurement. Patients about to get a CT scan are required to fast as well.
- Political application. Ever since, fasting is one tool that is used by political leaders and protesters to air out their protest, political statement or even awareness for a cause. This is often known as "hunger strike", a nonviolent method of resistance

practiced by participants where they fast as an act of political protest or to achieve awareness or goal for change. The most noteworthy events include the fasting of Gandhi and that had significant impact on the British Raj and the Indian population. In history, one "hunger strike" resulted in the death of 10 persons. It is in Northern Ireland in 1981, that a prisoner, Bobby Sands, was part of the 1981 Irish hunger strike, protesting for better rights in prison. Sands had just been elected to the British Parliament and died after 66 days of not eating. His funeral was attended by 100,000 people and the strike ended only after 9 other men died. In all, the ten men survived without food for 46 to 73 days taking only water and salt.

**Fast facts about Fasting**

In an excerpt from the book "Fasting to Freedom", the author discusses the effects of fasting and what is being eliminated in the process. Here we are given an overview as to how fasting works and its effect on us. Its been said that the other health benefits include stress resistance, increased insulin sensitivity, reduced morbidity, and increased life span

*"During a fast, a metamorphosis occurs. The body undergoes a tearing down and rebuilding of damaged materials. There is a remarkable redistribution of nutrients in the fasting body. It hangs on to precious minerals and vitamins while catabolising old tissue, toxins and inferior materials. The end result is a thorough cleansing of the tube, membrane and cellular structures. This process of cleansing and rebuilding has made fasting famous for its ability to rejuvenate, heal disease and give the body a more youthful tone.*

***Eliminations during the cleansing process***

- *Dead, dying or diseased cell*
  *Unwanted fatty tissue*
- *Trans-fatty acids*
- *Hardened coating of mucus on the intestinal wall*
- *Toxic waste matter in the lymphatic system and bloodstream*
- *Toxins in the spleen, liver and kidneys*
- *Mucus from the lungs and sinuses*
- *Imbedded toxins in the cellular fibres and deeper organ tissues*
- *Deposits in the microscopic tubes responsible for nourishing brain cells*
- *Excess cholesterol.*

*The Result*

- *Mental clarity is improved*
- *Rapid, safe weight loss is achieved without flabbiness*
- *The nervous system is balanced*
- *Energy level is increased*
- *Organs are revitalized*
- *Cellular biochemistry is harmonized*
- *The skin becomes silky, soft and sensitive*
- *There is greater ease of movement*
- *Breathing becomes fuller, freer and deeper*
- *The digestive system is given a well-deserved rest.*

*To heal illness, the body must pull all of its resources toward cleansing and repairing by removing appetite and reducing or stopping digestion. Wounded animals will fast, emerging to eat only after their wounds or broken bones have healed. This is the reason why there is little desire to eat food when sick—the body wants to focus all of its resources on cleansing."*

## Fasting our soul, body and mind.

Most of the experts on the field, fitness experts, doctors and spiritual experts, would agree as to the effects of fast on the soul and our body. Most striking is the article written by Gabrielle Lim when she summarized the benefits into five simple yet unforgettable sentences. In an excerpt from the article, she gives the 5 benefits.

### 1. Retune your digestive system

*Not many people know this but fasting can be a way for you to **give your digestive system a tune up.** According to Dr. Naomi Neufeld, an endocrinologist at UCLA, "You re-tune the body, suppress insulin secretion, reduce the taste for sugar, so sugar becomes something you're less fond of taking."*

*What happens is that the body eventually uses up the stored sugar (glycogen) so that less insulin is needed to help the body digest food. And that gives your pancreas a rest.*

### 2. Reduce your intake of free radicals

*Mark Mattson, a scientist with the National Institute on Aging, has reported that fasting can **reduce your intake of free radicals,** which can cause cancer. In fact, according to Mattson, "These free radicals will attack proteins, DNA, the nucleus* *of cells, the membranes of cells. They can damage all those different molecules in cells."*

*Even just reducing your calorie intake can have the same effects as a fast. In a study amongst rats and mice, it was noted that those who were fed very little and restricted in their food intake had a reduction in disease compared to those who were fed normal daily diets.*

### 3. Speed up your journey to self-discovery

*We are all creatures of habit. And eating, just like smoking and sleeping, is a habit. What happens during a fast is that by taking away such an essential part of your daily routine, you **mess up your whole schedule**. This sounds bad but it's not. It's really a time to reflect on your routines and give you a pause to think about how you want your life to move forward.*

*By fasting, you become more conscious of yourself and you can take the time usually spent eating to meditate, journal, or do any other form of reflection.*

### 4. Increase your gratitude

*How could you not be grateful to break your fast? And after each day when you do breakfast, it's a celebration. It is a celebration for a completed day of fasting, reflection, and persistence. **So rejoice and celebrate your success!** Show gratitude to yourself and others.*

*And when you break your fast, you will be very happy to taste food again. And contrary to some beliefs, you won't binge on food. In fact, you will be more conscious of what you allow into your body and **feel gratitude for the food you receive.***

### 5. Launch yourself into your ideal life

*Sounds like a pretty big benefit for something as simple as fasting. But it's true. When you begin your fast you can take this time to break old patterns, examine your current situation, and use it as the starting point for a whole new life.*

**Kinds of fasting**

Fasting can be done in many different ways. Below is a list of the different types or categories of fasting that is commonly practiced.

- Complete Fast: In complete fast, every two hours you drink a glass of water and a glass of warm water together with some lemon juice is taken an hour after. The main purpose of taking lemon juice in warm water is to prevent gas formation. If one needs some energy during this period, then a spoon of honey may also be taken with lemon juice in ordinary water also. Water of a tender coconut may also be taken during this fasting.

- Milk-Banana diet- In his kind of fast, one cup of skimmed milk and a banana is taken alternatively three to four times a day. Added to that honey and lemon juice and lemon juice in warm water may also be taken.

- Fruit diet: In this kind of fast, a person lives only on fruit and fruit juices. Again, in this fast, water and lemon juice in water can be continued. But his fast must not exceed 6-7 days; otherwise the body will become deficient of essential enzymes and amino acids.

- Fruit and Vegetable diet: In such a diet, lightly boiled or steamed vegetables can also be taken besides fruits. But the use of salt must be avoided. This fast can also not exceed more than 6-7 days at a stretch.

- Traditional Fast: In this kind of fast, a light meal is taken only once a day. This meal may contain a little of salt, sugar and fat. But one does not take any fruit, vegetables, tea, juices besides that meal. Ordinary water or lemon juice in warm water may be taken alternatively. This kind of fast is traditionally kept on full moon day or on the first day of the solar month.

- Water Fast: You can fast from 1 to 40 days. Try to drink 2 litres of water or more per day. The ten day water fast has become a recommended number of days. Ten days on water will cause the same weight loss as 30 days on juice. But water fasting is far more difficult, especially if you have a fast metabolism. Water fasting cleanses the body aggressively removing toxins rapidly. Water fasting can be more beneficial than juice fasting in combating more persistent forms of cancer, cleansing the tissues more aggressively. Water fasting demands mental preparation, the less pressure and responsibility you have during water fast the better. Think of it a holiday away form the normal patterns of living. Some recommend that the week before your fast, you drink fresh juices and eat mostly raw fruits and vegetables to cleanse the body so that the detoxification during water fasting will be less aggressive. Water fasting should always include two of three days of juice fasting before and after the water fast. This alternating between juice and water fasting is the most effective method of achieving a full cleansing through fasting.

- Juice fast: Juice fasting is safe and can allow the body to clean itself of toxins while greatly improving conditions for health. A benefit is that your energy level is high because you are receiving sufficient nutrients from the juices, so you can carry out normal activities. A juice fast takes some burden off the digestive system and frees up some energy for accelerated healing though water fast does much better in that regard. Also, juices can make available extra quantities of nutrients that a person might lack. Juices are easy to assimilate and take hardly any digestive energy from the body, allowing the body to put more energy into healing and rejuvenation. Packed with vitamins, minerals, living enzymes, antioxidants, photochemical, yet low enough in calories to force the body to cannibalize on its filthy waste, propelling you to vigorous physical health and clarity of mind.

## Preparing to fast

Depending on the length of your planned fast it can be helpful to prepare yourself for the change and the challenges you are about to face.

It is always better to inform yourself about fasting. Try doing your own investigation, read as much as you can on the fasting process, what are the various kinds of fasts and what you can expect as side effects. Never go into fasting if you have a pre-existing health condition. Consult your doctor if there are contrary indications with fasting and your condition.

Now, if it's your first time to fast and have not done any fasting before, start by doing things in smaller scale. Try doing it for, lets say2-3 hours or half-day. When you decide to do it in the evening, try going to sleep without eating or the whole morning on fasting. Do immediately try the whole day fast or 1 week fast as your body will be overwhelmed with the new situation.

Try to eat one single meal a day. The preparation should also include selection of what you will be eating. It is important to abstain from something that you always like pork or beef. Try to slowly cut-down your caffeine, alcohol or smoking routine for the following days. If you're a little bolder try to eat nothing but fruits and vegetables for a set amount of time. Whatever kind of test you can set up for yourself will give you an idea of what you will face once you jump fully into a more complete fast.

Most would agree that fasting detoxifies your body. By eating less or nothing at all your body has an opportunity to clean itself in a way it normally cannot.

Fasting is useless diet still consists of a lot of meat, processed foods, and you drink coffee and smoke. Sudden caffeine withdrawal can induce headaches if you are used to having caffeine every day. Cutting back or altering your diet days before you fast can help your body's detoxification process be less of a shock once you get into your fast.

Everyone would agree with what one expert on fasting said, *"Determine your cleanse duration and time period: Try to arrange that your fast is in a time period where you have low activity or lobsters. Avoid heavy kinds of work if at all possible. When it comes to long fasts and inability of somebody to handle a long fast, you just do the best you can. When detoxification increases as it does during fasting, the liver, kidneys, lungs and immune system work extra hard to handle the load."* As the purpose of the preparation is not to shock and overwhelm your body with fasting.

## Stages of fasting

Below is an excerpt from the book "How and When to Be Your Own Doctor" book, by Dr. Isabelle A. Moser with Steve Solomon, published in 1997. It clearly described the stages of fasting and how they work in relation to our body.

*The best way to understand what happens when we fast is to break up the process into six stages: preparation for the fast, loss of hunger, acidosis, normalization, healing, and breaking the fast.*

*A person that has consumed the typical American diet most of their life and whose life is not in immediate danger would be very wise to gently prepare their body for the fast. Two weeks would be a minimum amount of time, and if the prospective faster wants an easier time of it, they should allow a month or even two for preliminary housecleaning During this time, eliminate all meat, fish, dairy products, eggs, coffee, black tea, salt, sugar, alcohol, drugs, cigarettes, and greasy foods. This de-addiction will make the process of fasting much more pleasant, and is strongly recommended. However, eliminating all these harmful substances is withdrawal from addictive substances and will not be easy for most. I have more to say about this later when I talk about allergies and addictions.*

*The second stage, psychological hunger, usually is felt as an intense desire for food. This passes within three or four days of not eating anything. Psychological hunger usually begins with the first missed meal. If the faster seems to be losing their resolve, I have them drink unlimited quantities of good-tasting herb teas, (sweetened --only if absolutely necessary--with NutraSweet). Salt-free broths made from meatless instant powder (obtainable at the health food store) can also fend off the desire to eat until the stage of hunger has passed.*

*Acidosis, the third stage, usually begins a couple of days after the last meal and lasts about one week. During acidosis the body vigorously throws off acid waste products. Most people starting a fast begin with an overly acid blood pH from the typical American diet that contains a predominance of acid-forming foods. Switching over to burning fat for fuel triggers the release of even more acidic substances. Acidosis is usually accompanied by fatigue, blurred vision, and possibly dizziness. The breath smells very bad, the tongue is coated with bad-tasting dryish mucus, and the urine may be concentrated and foul unless a good deal of water is taken daily. Two to three quarts a day is a reasonable amount.*

*Most fasters feel much more comfortable by the end of the first seven to ten days, when they enter the normalization phase; here the acidic blood chemistry is gradually corrected. This sets the stage for serious healing of body tissues and organs. Normalization may take one or two more weeks depending on how badly the body was out of balance. As the blood chemistry steadily approaches perfection, the faster usually feels an increasing sense of well-being, broken by short spells of discomfort that are usually healing crises or retracing.*

*The next stage, accelerated healing, can take one or many weeks more, again depending on how badly the body has been damaged. Healing proceeds rapidly after the blood chemistry has been stabilized, the person is usually in a state of profound rest and the maximum amount of vital force can be directed toward repair and regeneration of tissues. This is a miraculous time when tumors are metabolized as food for the body, when arthritic deposits dissolve, when scar tissues tend to disappear, when damaged organs regain lost function (if they can). Seriously ill people who never fast long enough to get into this stage (usually it takes about ten days to two weeks of water fasting to seriously begin healing) never find out what fasting can really do for them.*

*Breaking the fast is equally or more important a stage than the fast itself. It is the most dangerous time in the entire fast. If you stop fasting prematurely, that is, before the body has completed detoxification and healing, expect the body to reject food when you try to make it eat, even if you introduce foods very gradually. The faster, the spiritual being running the body, may have become bored and want some action, but the faster's body hasn't finished. The body wants to continue healing.*

**Fasting for healing the body**

One of the most wanted benefits of fasting is the healing process that begins in the body during the fast. The healing process is said to happen when the body is searching for energy resources. When fasting, a fast energy is said to be diverted from the digestive system to another system, like the immune system, due to its lack of use.

Properly carried out, fasting can promote healing, is rejuvenating and can prolong one's life. Fasting is actually all about healing the body, unlike the conventional and alternative medicine. Ron Laguequist in his book pointed out that healing could be achieved through fasting.

He said that, *"Fasting intensifies healing as deep tissue and tired organs are repaired rapidly. To heal illness the body must pull all of its resources toward cleansing and repairing by removing appetite and reducing or stopping digestion. Wounded animals will fast, emerging to eat only after their injury or broken bones have healed. There are testimonies of people's old wounds aching during a fast for the first time in years; unnecessary scare tissue is being broken down as fuel. This is the reason why there is little desire to eat food when sick—the body wants to focus all of its resources on healing.*

*Why does fasting have such a powerful effect on healing the body? In the fasting state, the body scours for dead cells, damaged tissues, fatty deposits, tumors and abscesses, all of which are burned for fuel or expelled as waste. Diseased cells are dissolved in a systematic manner, leaving healthy tissue. The result is a thorough cleansing of the tubes, membranes and cellular structures. Ingestion of mucus-forming foods clogs the body's microscopic tubes and membranes, all of which are the highways used by the immune system. Fasting dissolves this internal mucus. During a fast it is common for the nose, throat and ears to pass sticky mucus, clogging the sinuses. Strands of mucus may be found in the stool after the first bowel movement. There is a remarkable redistribution of nutrients in the fasting body. It hangs on to precious minerals and vitamins while catabolizing on old tissue, toxins and inferior materials".*

**Fast the healthy way**

After knowing the benefits from fasting, keep in mind that when fasting, it should always be the healthy way. Do not fast for the sake that it's the trend or because you want look sexy because others are. It should be holistic and beneficial to you and your outlook.

So, how do you fast the healthy way?

1. Be accountable. Whatever the consequences are, be accountable for your actions and for other things. Likewise, be sensitive to the response or reaction of others towards your fasting. They might have seen something wrong with your fasting.

2. Prepare in advance. When you want to fast, do not act on impulse, it best to be prepared. Try to know what could be things that might actually happen before, during and after the fast. It is always safe to prepare in advance the things you are about to do. The time of transition is useful for the body, but can also be used to prepare on spiritual and practical levels as well. If you don't skimp on the preparation time, your fast will likely go more smoothly and be more effective.

3. Understand the effects on your body. Your body goes through several distinct phases when you begin to fast. It is possible that during the first few hours, you will feel weak. Don't be alarmed yet as this is natural since your body begins to eliminate the toxins in your system. There are a lot more of things that will happen but again, don't be alarmed as they are normal and will disappear as soon your fasting is over.

4. Break the fast properly. The body through a period of heightened detoxification. An extended fast should have medical guidance that includes plans on how to deal with some potentially serious issues once your fast ends. The body has adjusted to a different state and must not be severely shock it by eating and drinking things that will cause discomfort and physical problems.

**Who should not fast?**

Fasting, no matter how properly it is done, will always have dangerous effects on certain people. It is best advised that these should not fast even if they want to. Here are the categories of people who should never fast or must practice extreme caution.

1. Infants and children. There is really no reason for infants and children to fast. Due to their lack of maturity, they would likely not really understand the spiritual purpose of fasting, and their bodies need to take in ample nutrients regularly.

2. Pregnant women. Water-only fasts should definitely be avoided by women who are pregnant or nursing. The baby requires so many nutrients for normal development and is dependent on the mother's proper nutrition to receive those nutrients. You are forcing the unborn baby to fast as well if the mother decides to fast.

3. People with cancer. Cancer is usually indicative of, among other things, an immune system that is not in good shape.

4. People with other health concerns. Water-only fasts should be avoided by those with significant health issues such as diabetes. However, juice fasts MAY be an option, but should be undertaken only under a doctor's close supervision.

5. The elderly. Water-only fasts should be avoided by elderly people. There is no need for the elderly to fast as their body may not be able to carry such task.

And if one has still some concerns or questions, they should always ask with their doctor. Remember, fasting is supposed to bring out the best and healthy us.

**Tips on fasting**

Here are some fasting tips shared by Debopriya Bose

*For those who do not fast regularly or are doing it for the first time, it is better to adopt a moderate approach towards fasting and then graduate to stricter regimes. Start with a 1-day program. Then move on to programs for 2 days, 3 days and so on. In between the fasting days, one can have food consisting of raw fruits, vegetables, soups and juices. This is a good way of*
*Graduating to 5 or 10 days fast.*

*A first timer could consider juice fasting than water fasting as juice fasting is easier than water fast. Also juice fast provides most of the nutrients and calories that solid foods provide. Hence one would not miss solid food when on a juice fast.*

*One of the important fasting tips is to prepare the body slowly for the process. For beginners, it is helpful to start fasting with a little bit of food each day. Extend the fast to 12 to 14 hours in the evening (including sleep). Such a method could also be adopted for a couple of days before actually starting the fast. For greater benefits from fasting, one should stop the intake of alcohol, caffeine, red meat, sugar and poultry for a few days before going in for a fast. Also, the intake of nutritional supplements should be limited. Natural is the way to go during fasting!*
*For the first 2 days one may feel irritated and experience headaches. However, from the 3rd day onwards, one's body adjusts better to the fasting program. To avoid such symptoms, one could take a meal that would comprise of water, juices, tea or snacks made from fresh fruits and vegetables, sometime around 3 p.m.*

*As it is clear that even during fasting, all the nutritional requirements of the body are met; there is no reason to stop working out. In fact regular exercise will help expedite the cleansing process. However, beginners can go easy with their workouts in case they are used to heavy workouts. Yoga and meditation are great ways to complement the healing process during fasting.*

*One of the important tips for fasting is not to start binging on food once you are out of it. Since the body has already got accustomed to eating healthy and only as much as required, fasting is good opportunity to start off with healthy eating habits.*

*Those who are underweight or pregnant should not fast. People who have undergone a surgery or are suffering from anemia, hyperglycemia, and chronic problems of heart, kidneys or lungs should avoid going on a fast. Nevertheless, if one is suffering from some health condition it is always better to consult a physician before starting a fast.*

*Fasting is not a crash course for weight loss. Despite all the benefits, listen to your body. If one feels ill while fasting, call in the doctor. It is important to follow the fasting tips in order to reap the benefits of fasting that ensures overall wellbeing of the body.*

## Sample fasting program for starters

Now that you pretty much know about fasting and its benefits, try this simple fasting regime using fruit juice.

1. Begin by clearing out any junk food from your home if you intend to do even a short 2 or 3-day juice fast. Having cookies and potato chips nearby in your kitchen while you juice fast will require enormous will power to refrain from eating them. You can give these items to a friend to store until you complete your juice fast or simply donate them to your local soup kitchen.
2. Purchase organic fruits and vegetables from your local farmer's markets or the health food store. If you purchase non-organic produce, avoid buying grapes, apples, or peaches as these items are generally grown with heavy pesticide
3. Make a detox bath for non-organic produce by filling a large tub with filtered water and 2 teaspoons of Clorox bleach. Submerge the non-organic produce only in this bleach bath for 15 minutes. Rinse thoroughly and drain.
4. Juice fasting requires you chop, cut and peel assorted vegetables and fruits before you juice them through a heavy-duty juicer so that you are consuming the vitamins and minerals immediately. There is quite a difference between canned fruit juice and freshly prepared juices. Storing fresh juices in your refrigerator for 4 to 5 hours is acceptable but avoid doing so overnight.
5. Combining fruits and vegetables is generally okay but there are certain combinations that may be hard to digest or are simply not palatable. A classic rule of thumb was that apples of all types can be juiced with any other fruit and vegetable as apples will digest easily for most people. Melons are best eaten alone. Melons tend to digest very quickly and if consumed with other foods, you

may experience indigestion of the foods or liquids that take the body more time to digest. Common sense and personal taste preference will guide you. For example, juicing carrots and bananas and kale together will probably not yield a juice you will enjoy.

6.  Juicing basics: prepare only as much as you will need to consume at each setting. For example, a good snacking juice is made from juicing 2 apples, 1 small carrot, one half of a small lemon and ½ teaspoon of gingerroot. For an excellent breakfast juice, combine ½ large medjool date (for the date sugar), 1 medium banana, liquid from a coconut (or to cheat, use "lite" coconut milk from a can, if diluted 1 part coconut milk to 3 parts filtered water), adding filtered water to thin to your desired consistency.

7.  Juicing for lunch or dinner drinks could include combinations any vegetable with apples to sweeten. For example, juice 5 to 6 large leaves of curly kale (or lacinto or dinosaur kale), ½ cup parsley, 2 stalks of celery, 1 large carrot and ½ teaspoon of gingerroot or cayenne pepper. Try 6 leaves of rainbow chard, 6 leaves of baby bokchoy, beets (the tops as well), and a very small bulb of garlic for a spicy dinner drink.

8.  Drink at least 6 to 8, 8-ounce glasses of filtered water to help you adjust to the cleansing effects of juice fasting. If you intend to juice fast for more than a day, add 1 tablespoon ground flax seeds to any drink and consume three times a day to make certain you are moving your bowels in the absence of soluble and insoluble fiber (as is found in the skins and cellulose of vegetables.)

9.  Do not be ambitious while juice fasting. Do not starve yourself by consuming too few juice drinks. Prepare from scratch and consume at least 5 to 6 fresh juice drinks in any 24-hour period along with the 6 to 8 glasses of filtered water.

10. If you find that after the first 6 hours of such a juice fast you experience any changes in heart rate (very rapid or slower than normal), dizziness, headaches, or extreme physical fatigue, consider limiting your juicing to only that 6-hour time frame. For example, juice Friday morning until noon. If you are miserable, consider breaking the fast gently with steamed vegetables, vegetable soup, plain toast and unsweetened organic yogurt. Do not break your juice fast with a steak and fries or a pizza.

11. Depending on your general health prior to juice fasting, it is common to experience headaches and several additional bowel movements as your body begins to cleanse. Transition slowly back to solid foods by introducing steamed vegetables, easy-to-digest proteins such as scrambled eggs, yogurt, or chicken soup.

12. Break the juice fast slowly so that you are not overwhelming your digestive system. If you experience what is called a "healing crisis" and find the juice fast kicks off a flu or minor cold bring

your juice fast slowly to a close, adding vegetable and chicken soups back into your diet slowly. Rest as needed and cut back on very strenuous exercise while juicing.

## Conclusion

There are lot of things to know more about fasting. As we age, we hear so much about fasting that we don't know which are real and which are not.   But there are many reasons to consider fasting as a benefit to one's health. The body is one amazing thing as rids itself of the toxins that have built up in our fat stores throughout the years. It also heals itself, repairs all the damaged organs during a fast. And finally, there is good evidence to show that regulated fasting contributes to longer life.

Yet many doctors warn against fasting for extended periods of time without supervision. There are still many doctors today who deny all of these points and claim that fasting is detrimental to one's health and have evidence to back their statements. That is because fasting is still considered to be as just the simple deprivation of the body the much-needed food. The idea of depriving a body of what society has come to view as so essential to our survival in order to heal continues to be a topic of controversy.

Let us not forget however that the effectiveness of the fasting we do still depend on ourselves. How we look at fasting and why we fast will still play a major role in determining the success of the fasting we just did.

All in all, the reason we fast may be about weight reduction, health improvement, or healing of the body. Regardless of the reason, fasting should be not be scary and what's important is that we enjoy and relax ourselves as we fast. It should be a meaningful experience for us.

So, better pick up that pen and plan away to healthy, new you!

# PART 4

# SECRET FOOD COMBINATIONS

# Table of contents



## Introduction

If ever there is one universal language, it would definitely be food. As the years go by, we try to understand and reconcile ourselves with the power of food over our lives. They could make us young or old, fat or slim, health or weak. Because of this, a lot of studies and discoveries were made on the topic of food.

As well look at us in the mirror, most of us would almost immediately notice those lines in our faces. Suddenly we all wonder if we are too old or the environment around us is simply moving time so fast. We wonder what could be done.

When we got up and stepped on that scale, we are shocked to see that line hit past the average weight. We panic as we think that we are getting fat and would mean getting slow. Mentally we relate our weight to our heavy bodies and low energy. We almost immediately sign up for that gym class.

We are extremely conscious of what we look that we tend to forgot that sometimes the answer could be that simple. In our society today, we are bombarded with pollutions and fast food. These two have a tremendous effect on how we eat and look. Fast food centres offer unhealthy food that often times contribute a lot of problems.

Lots of studies and experiments are being done to answer our cry for help. We want a diet that is effective. A diet that could boost our energy levels, make us feel young, look young, affordable and sustainable.

One interesting and very realistic discovery is "food combining". Correctly combining foods makes all the difference in the world to proper digestion, cholesterol and metabolism. Without complete digestion, the nutrients in even the most wholesome food cannot be fully extracted and assimilated by the body.

Before we could even say or open our mouth bout food combining, we must first be equipped with the basic knowledge about food, its classifications and digestion. We cannot disregard these as they are the fundamental stones of which this was based. Thus in the chapters below there are some review on the basic data to fully grasp and understand the concept of food combining.

Let's us remember this word of wisdom before we begin.

*Food and drink are relied upon to nurture life. But if one does not know that the nature of substances may be opposed to each other, and one consumes them altogether indiscriminately, the vital organs will be thrown out of harmony and disastrous consequences will soon arise. Therefore, those who wish to nurture their lives must carefully avoid doing such damage to them.*

*[Chia Ming, Essential Knowledge for Eating and Drinking, 1368 AD].*

## Food and nutrition

It must not be forgotten that nutrition begins with food. The science of nutrition is related almost to everything with the body that does with food in order to function, live, heal and grow. Food is any substance, composed of carbohydrates, water, fats and/or proteins, that is either eaten or drunk by any animal, including humans, for nutrition or pleasure. Items considered food may be sourced from plants, animals or other categories such as fungus. Although many human cultures sought food items through hunting and gathering, today most cultures use farming, ranching, and fishing, with hunting, foraging and other methods of a local nature included but playing a minor role.

Now foods that are eaten on a regular basis are called diet. And every single person has its own unique diet. The geographic location and family traditions play extremely major parts in the formation of a person's diet although as the person grows, the diet may change but to a little degree. Food choices vary from people to people just as they vary with almost every living creature.

We cannot make our own food out from the sun or from the wind of from the water. Our food comes from the plants, which make their food, and from animals that are pretty much like us dependent on plants. The plants, with the help of the sun, make their food form the chemicals found in water, air and soil. Animals eat their food, or feed, raw since they are equipped with specialized digestive organs, perfected through evolution to digest the food they eat.

On the other hand, we humans eat both plants and animals. We like to prepare our food and in most countries, food preparation is an art that takes years to perfect. Different countries have different staple foods. Mostly in Asia, rice and corn are ever present in the table. In western countries, potato and bread are their staple food. Regardless of the difference, these staple foods are the major source of carbohydrates. Protein and milk are likewise present in the table. Only people are too busy gobbling down their food that they don't care about the food they are eating or its nutritional value. It is vital that proteins, carbohydrate and fats are present. The function of these will be discussed in the succeeding chapters.

We must never attempt to skip a meal for the sake of weight loss. The more we deprive ourselves with food, the worse our body will become. Our conditions will worsen even if physically we look great.

**Importance of food**

We cannot deny the fact that we need food in order to survive. Food and water has been the centre of our life. Humans can survive without their big houses, expensive cars and clothes but they could never survive for more than a week without any food and water.

If you could observe, large parts of the third world countries suffer from malnutrition. They have food but the foods they have do not meet the daily required calories or energy of the body. Also, they do not have enough food for the day that they could only eat once or twice a day. As they say, "you are what you eat". If we eat all those greasy and oily foods, we tend to become overweight or unhealthy. If we eat only sweets and caffeine, then don't expect that we could have that perfect, healthy body we always dream.

So just how important is the food?

- Food is our primary source of energy. We need energy for our everyday activities which starts the moment we open our eyes in the morning.

- As energy source, they are the ones responsible for our growing process, rebuilding of damaged cells and regulation of body systems.

- Food also produces heat in the form of energy.

- Food makes us healthy and strong. This includes our immune system. A vital system that acts our defence against disease and sickness.

- Food makes us glow and young looking. A well nourished person looks young for his or her age as her body is able to deal with the daily stress it faces.

To function properly, the human body must have nutrients that are present in the food.  Our brain cannot function if the body is weak. We will suffer from fatigue and stress from the lack of food. Extreme dieting is harmful to us and our body. Our digestive system and our cardio-vascular system are the ones at greatest risk to being damaged and become not repairable.

**Food Pyramid**

The basic four food groups were reworked into a more balanced and healthy food pyramid guide. Now this food pyramid has its base on the grain group, the second level with fruit and vegetables group, third level with meat and diary groups and on the last level, fats, oils and sweets group.

The food pyramid is generally a guide for everyone of what to be eaten each and as to how much quantity should be eaten. There should be a variety and balance in eating so as to meet the required calories per day. Each group provides what a person needs but in small amounts. No food group in the food pyramid could provide all the nutrients that a person needs. Also, the foods in the pyramids have no substitute and must not be replaced by any commercial products stating that they are the substitute.

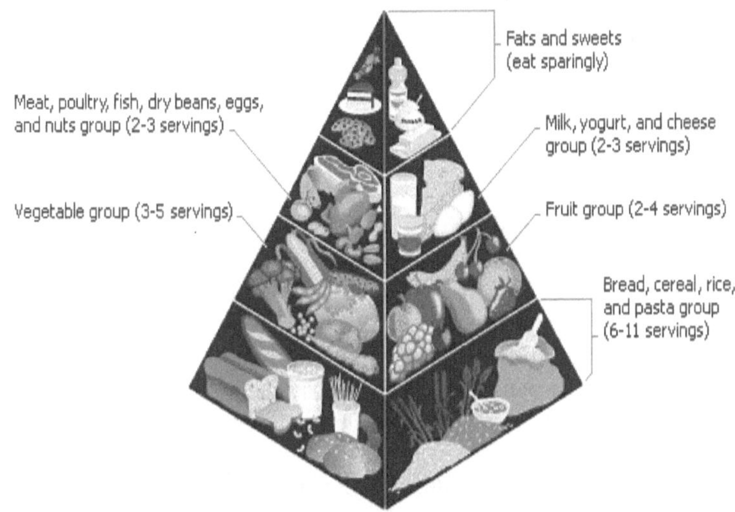



The grain group which is found at the base of the pyramid is composed mainly of cereals, pasta, rice and other foods made from grains. We need a lot of daily servings of these foods than any other groups because they are our source of B-vitamins, iron, carbohydrates and some protein. The daily recommendation is at least 6 servings per day.

Fruit and vegetable group are the richest source of vitamins and minerals. Take note, they provide fiber which may not contain nutrients but is extremely important for the digestive system. They aide in the smooth digestion of the food and thus ensure good digestion. At least 3-5 serving so f vegetables and 2-4 serving of fruits per day is recommended.

Meat and diary groups are the richest source of proteins. On this level, the two groups of food such as milk, fish, eggs, poultry and cheese are all animal source except for nuts and beans which are from plants. High amounts of protein, calcium, iron, phosphorus, zinc and B vitamins. These are essential in bone and muscle development which why children need more meat and dairy products in their diet during their growing years.

Fats, oils and sweets group are on the top of the pyramid and is recommended to be used sparingly. Even if they are a pleasure to eat, they provide only calories and very little nutrients to our body. These include cream, chocolates, sugars, candy sodas and cakes. Too much of this results in have ailments and problems with the heart and blood sugar.

**Malnutrition**

It is likewise important to know what malnutrition is. This will be vital as some weight loss diet deprive our body with the much-needed nutrients and lead to malnutrition without our knowledge.

So, what is malnutrition? It is the imbalance between the body's demand for nutrition and the available supply of nutrients. When the body is not given enough of any of the essential nutrients over a certain period of time, it will result to becoming weak and more prone to infection and sickness. The body withers as a result of the muscle being broken down for energy since the body will tap its stored fats for energy. In extreme cases, death occurs.

What causes it then? It can result from an unsatisfactory diet that often results to starvation oneself by force. It can likewise come from a disorder that interferes with the body's utilization of food.

But did you know that obesity is also a form of malnutrition? It is being defined as body weight more than 20 percent above the ideal body weight.

Extreme weight loss such as that in anorexics is life-threatening. It is one form of malnutrition that is extremely rampant among women. Anorexia nervosa is condition that requires professional treatment and emotional support from family and friends.

In unindustrialized countries, protein-calorie malnutrition is one problem that is common among children. Their bodies fail to grow with damage digestive organs. Starvation results in calorie deficiency.

Lack of the critical nutrients results in the deficiency of vitamins and minerals that are responsible for different disorders. Like, lack of iron results to anemia, lack of iodine results to goiter which is the enlargement of the thyroid gland and many other diseases detrimental to the body.

**How the digestive system works**

The foods we eat are not in a form that the body can use as nourishment. Food and drink must be changed into smaller molecules of nutrients before they can be absorbed into the blood and carried to cells throughout the body. Digestion is the process by which food and drink are broken down into their smallest parts so the body can use them to build and nourish cells and to provide energy.

Digestion involves mixing food with digestive juices, moving it through the digestive tract, and breaking down large molecules of food into smaller molecules. Digestion begins in the mouth, when we chew and swallow, and is completed in the small intestine.

So how does digestion work?

Well, the large, hollow organs of the digestive tract contain a layer of muscle that enables their walls to move. The movement of organ walls can propel food and liquid through the system and also can mix the contents within each organ. Food moves from one organ to the next through muscle action called peristalsis. Peristalsis looks like an ocean wave travelling through the muscle. The muscle of the organ contracts to create a narrowing and then propels the narrowed portion slowly down the length of the organ.

These waves of narrowing push the food and fluid in front of them through each hollow organ.

The first major muscle movement occurs when food or liquid is swallowed. Although we are able to start swallowing by choice, once the swallow begins, it becomes involuntary and proceeds under the control of the nerves.

Swallowed food is pushed into the esophagus, which connects the throat above with the stomach below. At the junction of the esophagus and stomach, there is a ring like muscle, called the lower esophageal sphincter, closing the passage between the two organs. As food approaches the closed sphincter, the sphincter relaxes and allows the food to pass through to the stomach.

The stomach has three mechanical tasks. First, it stores the swallowed food and liquid. To do this, the muscle of the upper part of the stomach relaxes to accept large volumes of swallowed material. The second job is to mix up the food, liquid, and digestive juice produced by the stomach. The lower part of the stomach mixes these materials by its muscle action. The third task of the stomach is to empty its contents slowly into the small intestine.

Several factors affect emptying of the stomach, including the kind of food and the degree of muscle action of the emptying stomach and the small intestine. Carbohydrates, for example, spend the least amount of time in the stomach, while protein stays in the stomach longer, and fats the longest. As the food dissolves into the juices from the pancreas, liver, and intestine, the contents of the intestine are mixed and pushed forward to allow further digestion.

Finally, the digested nutrients are absorbed through the intestinal walls and transported throughout the body. The waste products of this process include undigested parts of the food, known as fiber, and older cells that have been shed from the mucosa. These materials are pushed into the colon, where they remain until the feces are expelled by a bowel movement.


**Importance of digestion**
Most digested molecules of food are absorbed through the small intestine. They may either have been mechanically digested (food is chewed, mashed and broken down into smaller pieces) or chemically digested (enzymes change food into simpler substances).
So what makes digestion so important? Digestion is the breaking of food into smaller pieces so that it could be absorbed and utilized by our body. The smaller pieces that were broken down are then absorbed into the small intestine where they will be transported to the different body parts. The body in return utilizes for the nourishment of the cells and be an energy source. Like tiny building blocks, they work together to form

every part of you. Cells make up the skin, bones, muscles, and organs. Our body uses nutrients to fix damaged cells and make new ones. Nutrients give cells what they need to work, grow, and divide. Consider the foods we eat at the raw materials or ingredients of a dish. In order for us to be able to make a certain dish, the ingredients must chopped and processed so that they will fully utilized and cook. The same way goes with digestion.

Improper digestion results from the different digestive problems. This could also come from the mal-absorption of the different nutrients. Lets us not forget that our digestive system support our body. As small as we think that system is, we cannot overlook the fact its importance. It is composed of a series of organs that break down and absorb the food we eat so that the nutrients can be transported into the blood stream and delivered to cells throughout the body. Most of us ignore our digestive system unless there's a problem. We never or if not, rarely consider the role it plays in our overall health. To think, move, work, and learn, we need our digestive system to process your food and help utilize the nutrients. Our skin, hair, and even sleep can be affected by whether or not everything is working correctly.

One expert says that people with poor digestive health might struggle with their weight, experience irregularity, nausea, bloating, constipation, stomach pain, diarrhea, heartburn, or gas on a routine basis. Poor digestive health also can prevent people from sleeping, working, exercising, or socializing with friends.

So bear in mind that our digestive system affects our whole body when it is not well taken cared of.

**What's Food Combination?**

Food combining, or scientifically called, Trophology, is the science of correct food-combining, that is, the art of knowing which foods go best with which others. 'Food combining' may also mean to the combination of foods which are compatible with each other in terms of digestive chemistry. Food combining is a basic component of optimal nutrition because it allows the body to digest and utilize the nutrients in our foods to their full extent.

Most would agree that *"Food combining is based on the theory that different food groups require different digestion times. Digestion is helped the most by using foods which have roughly the same digestion time."* Thus, correct food combinations are important for proper digestion, utilization, and assimulation of the nutrients in our diet. The principles of food combining are dictated by digestive chemistry. Different foods require different digestive enzymes to aid in the digestive process - some acid, some alkaline.

Below is a list of foods and their digestion time.
- Water  when stomach is empty, leaves immediately and goes into intestines,
- Juices
    - Fruit vegetables, vegetable broth - 15 to 20 minutes.
- Semi-liquid
    - (blended salad, vegetables or fruits) - 20 to 30 min.
- Fruits
    - Watermelon - 20 min. digestion time.
      Other melons - Cantaloupes, Cranshaw, Honeydew etc. - 30 min.

Oranges, grapefruit, grapes - 30 min.

Apples, pears, peaches, cherries etc. - digest in 40 min.

- Vegetables
  - Raw tossed salad vegetables - tomato, lettuces, cucumber, celery, red or green pepper, and other succulent vegetables - 30 to 40 min. digestion. -
- Steamed or cooked vegetables
  - Leafy vegetables - escarole, spinach, kale, collards etc. - 40 min. - Zucchini, broccoli, cauliflower, string beans, yellow squash, and corn on cob - all 45 min. digestion time

    Root vegetables - carrots, beets, parsnips, and turnips etc. - 50 min.
- Semi-Concentrated Carbohydrates - Starches
  - Jerusalem artichokes & leafy, acorn & butternut squashes, corn, potatoes, sweet potatoes, yam, chestnuts - all 60 min. digestion.
- Concentrated Carbohydrates - Grains
  - Brown rice, millet, buckwheat, cornmeal, oats (first 3 vegetables best) - 90 min.
- Legumes & Beans - (Concentrated Carbohydrate & Protein)
  - Lentils, limas, chick peas, peas, pigeon peas, kidney beans, etc. - 90 min. digestion time

    soy beans -120 min. digestion time
- Seeds & Nuts
  - Seeds - Sunflower, pumpkin, pepita, sesame - Digestive time approx. 2 hours.

    Nuts - Almonds, filberts, peanuts (raw), cashews, brazil, walnuts, pecans etc. - 2 1/2 to 3 hours to digest.
- Dairy
  - Skim milk, cottage or low fat pot cheese or ricotta - approx. 90 min. digestion time

    whole milk cottage cheese - 120 min. digestion

    whole milk hard cheese - 4 to 5 hours digestion time
- Animal proteins
  - Egg yolk - 30 min. digestion time

    Whole egg - 45 min.

    Fish - cod, scrod, flounder, sole seafood - 30 min. digestion time

    Fish - salmon, salmon trout, herring, (more fatty fish) - 45 min. to 60 digestion time

    Chicken - 1½ to 2 hours digestion time (without skin)

    Turkey - 2 to 2 ¼ hours digestion time (without skin)

    Beef, lamb - 3 to 4 hours digestion time

    Pork - 4½ to 5 hours digestion time

## Dr. Hay and Food Combining

*"Any carbohydrate foods require alkaline conditions for their complete digestion, so must not be combined with acids of any kind, as sour fruits, because the acid will*

According to common story, when William Howard Hay (1866–1940) graduated from New York University Medical College in 1891, he practiced medicine and specialized in surgery. That changed 16 years later when his own medical troubles led him to research the connection between diet and health. Hay then weighed 225 pounds (102 kilograms) and had high blood pressure and Bright's disease, a kidney condition. Hay discovered that his heart was dilated while running to catch a train.

The dilated heart caused by weakened heart muscles meant that his blood could not pump efficiently. Hay knew from treating patients that his future did not "look overlong or very bright," according to his 1929 book *Health via Food*. The title described Hay's health theories, his condition, and treatment.

Hay diagnosed the causes of his conditions as the "very familiar trinity of troubles" that then ranked as the primary cause of death: the combination of high blood pressure, kidney disease, and dilated heart. But he could not accept the fact that his legs, which have swollen that time might be chopped off. So he looked for other reasons and so Hay looked at his eating habits.

Thus he went into research and it was said that, *Hay's research led to a diet based on the theory that health was affected by the chemical process of digestion. The body uses an alkaline digestive process for **carbohydrates**, the group that Hay classified as consisting of starchy foods and sweet things. The digestion of proteins involved acid. If carbohydrates and proteins were consumed at the same time, the alkaline process was interrupted by the acid process. Combining incompatible foods caused acidosis, the accumulation of excess acid in body fluids. Hay linked the combination of foods to medical conditions like Bright's disease and diabetes. The wrong combinations "drained vitality" and caused people to gain weight.*

*Hay maintained that the solution was to eat proteins at one meal and carbohydrates at another. He classified fruits with acids. Hay labelled vegetables in the neutral category that could be consumed with either group. He also advocated the daily administration of an enema to cleanse the colon.*

This was the starting point for the interest in the field by other doctors who would later have a classification of the food system.

**Food Sources**

- *Protein*

The principal sources of protein are:

1. Meats of all kinds (the lean part), such as beef, veal, mutton, lean pork, chicken, turkey, duck, goose, game, both feathered and furred, in fact, all lean flesh from animals and birds.

2. Fish of all kinds, such as trout, salmon, herring, pickerel, pike, cod, halibut, mackerel, sturgeon, and shad. Also shellfish, like oysters (which are mostly water), clams, crabs and lobsters.

3. Legumes, the chief of which are all kinds of dried beans, dried peas, lentils and peanuts. Also green peas, and both the green and the dried lima beans should be consumed.

4. Dairy products, including sweet milk, light milk, buttermilk, cottage cheese and all other kinds of cheese. Cream contains but little protein, and butters practically none.

5. Nuts, especially almonds, Brazil nuts, filberts, hickory nuts, pecans, English walnuts, butternuts, pistachios and pignolias. (Peanuts are legumes, not true nuts. Chestnuts contain much starch and only a little protein.)

- *Starchy or carbohydrates*

The chief sources of our starchy foods are:

1. Cereals, the most important being wheat of all kinds, Indian corn, rice, rye, barley, and oats. No matter in what form we eat them—in bread, toast, cakes, mushes, flaked or puffed cereals—they are starchy.

2. Tubers, the most important being Irish potatoes, sweet potatoes and Jerusalem artichoke. The dasheen is also a tuber, which resembles the white potato in consistency, and has an agreeable flavour.

3. Legumes, especially when they are ripe. The ripe limas, navy beans and other kinds of ripe beans, peas, lentils and peanuts are starchy. Green limas and young peas contain more starch than the other vegetables; usually classified as succulent.

4. Nuts, but only a few varieties. Acorns, dried chestnuts and cocoanuts are rich in starch.

- *Fats and oils*

The chief sources of our fats are:

1. Dairy products—cream, butter and some rich cheeses.

2. Flesh of dead animals, especially pork, mutton and beef, which have been fattened.

3. Fat fish, such as herring, shad and salmon trout.

4. Legumes. Some kinds of peanuts are very oily, and so are soy beans.

5. Nuts of nearly every kind. Almonds, Brazil nuts, filberts, hickory nuts, pecans, English walnuts, butternuts, cocoanuts, pistachios and acorns are rich in oil.

6. Cotton seed, olives, and corn furnish much edible oil.

- *Fruits*

Some of the most common juicy fruits are:

Apples, lemons, oranges, peaches, pears, strawberries, apricots, avocadoes, blackberries, cherries, cranberries, currants, gooseberries, grapes, huckleberries, blueberries, mulberries, nectarines, olives, pineapples, plums, raspberries and whortleberries.

The melons (watermelon, muskmelon, cantaloupe, casaba, honey dew, etc.), rhubarb stalk and tomatoes are so like fruit that for practical purposes we may call them so.

The most important sweet fruits are:

Ripe bananas, sweet prunes, sweet grapes, raisins, dried currants, figs, dates and persimmons

- *Succulent and salad vegetables*

The principal succulent vegetables are:

Asparagus, beets, cabbage, carrots, turnips, parsnips, cauliflower, cucumber, egg plant, lettuce, okra (gumbo), onions, radish, summer squash, tomatoes, spinach, kohlrabi, kale, Brussels sprouts, cone artichoke, chard, string beans, celery, turnip tops, lotus, endive, dandelion, oyster plant, rutabaga and garlic. Though corn is really a cereal, corn in the milk, either on the cob or canned and green peas may also be classed with the succulent vegetables and also the pumpkin.

The principal salad vegetables are:

Lettuce, celery, endive, romaine, chicory, tomatoes, cucumbers, cabbage, celery cabbage, parsley, field lettuce, and cress are suggested. All leaves that are relished may be used for salad purposes.

**The Nine Rules**

Food combining cannot be done without any rules. And it is dilated by the digestive system and the digestive process. This is as dictated as the different food types require different digestion length and process. It is then important that when doing food combining, do not just combine just because you think it is right. You must know the basics and what food goes well with another.

Dr. Herbert Shelton in his book" Combining Food Made Easy", gave some easy and simple combinations so as not to confuse a beginner or someone interested in the diet.

The Nine Basic Rules of Proper Food Combining:
- *Eat acids and starchy foods at separate meals. Acids neutralize the alkaline medium     required for starch digestion and the result is fermentation and indigestion.*
- *Eat food containing protein and carbohydrate at separate meals. Protein foods require an acid medium for digestion.*
- *Eat only one kind of protein food at a meal.*
- *Proteins and acid foods must be eaten at separate meals. The acids of acid foods inhibit the secretion of the digestive acids required for protein digestion. Undigested protein putrefies in bacterial decomposition and produces some potent poisons.*
- *Fatty foods and proteins should be eaten at separate meals. Some foods, especially nuts, are over 50% fat and require hours for digestion.*
- *Fruits contain natural sugar and proteins should be eaten at separate meals.*
- *Eat sugars (fruits) and starchy foods at separate meals. Fruits undergo no digestion in the stomach and are held up if eaten with foods that require digestion in the stomach.*
- *Eat melons alone. They do not combine with any other type of foods.*
- *Desserts should be eaten separately without combining with any other type of foods. Eaten on top of meals they lie heavy on the stomach, requiring no digestion there, and ferment. Bacteria turn them into alcohols and vinegars and acetic acids.*

**Food combination Table**

When having meals, it is better to take note that the smaller the number of courses, the better it will be. Food combining is not about the bulk or the quantity of food you eat but the quality and the combination observed in the meal. What is important is that the meals should be favourable to the well being and health of someone rather than the complexity of its preparation.

Proteins, fats and carbohydrates remain in our stomach for as long as seven hours until all the stomach contents empty. Depending on how they are paired with, carbohydrates pretty much have a short stay in the stomach when eaten alone without protein. Even shorter are the fruit meals while proteins have the longest stay in the stomach. So it is ideal that the three be eaten at different meals. Like for breakfast, you could opt for just a fruit meal or a protein meal with say like salad and vegetables when it comes to dinner. The choices are many as long as you know how to combine them. The rules are there to guide you.

Even more, the food combinations will be greatly aided by this chart.

Food Combining Chart

| Food Groups | Proteins | Fats | Starches | Vegetables | Sweet Fruits | Sub-acid Fruits | Acid Fruits |
|---|---|---|---|---|---|---|---|
| Proteins | Good | Poor | Poor | Good | Poor | Fair | Good |
| Fats | Poor | Good | Fair | Good | Fair | Fair | Fair |
| Starches | Poor | | Good | Good | Fair | Fair | Poor |
| Vegetables | Good | Good | Good | Good | Poor | Poor | Poor |
| Sweet Fruits | Poor | | Fair | Poor | Good | Good | Poor |
| Sub-acid Fruits | Fair | | Fair | Poor | Good | Good | Good |
| Acid Fruits | Good | | Poor | Poor | Poor | Good | Good |

- *Proteins:* Nuts, seeds, soya beans, cheese, eggs, poultry* meat*, fish*, yogurt.
- *Fats:* Oils, olive, butter, margarine.
- *Starches:* Whole cereals, peas, beans, lentils.

- *Vegetables:* Leafy green vegetables, sprouted seeds, cabbage cauliflower, broccoli, green peas, celery, tomatoes, onions.
- *Sweet Fruits:* Bananas, fits, custard apples, all-dried fruits, dates.
- *Sub-acid-fruits:* Grapes, pears, apples, peaches, apricots, plums, fruits guavas, raspberries.
- *Acid fruits:* Grapefruit, lemons, oranges, limes, pineapple, strawberries.

* Not recommended for good nutrition.

**Food combination-digestion pairing**

Writer Carly Schuna shares her thoughts about the topic. In her article, she discusses the relation of food combining and digestion. We must remember however that what might work for one person, may not hold true to another.

*"Food combining involves eating foods in certain combinations or sequences with the goal of aiding digestion and minimizing stomach discomfort. People who advocate food combining follow guidelines that dictate how to combine foods at meals and in what sequence to eat each food. They feel that improperly combined meals can result in digestive discomfort, a build up of food in the stomach and even more serious health problems.*

### *Digestion*

*A basic principle of food combining is to only combine foods that have similar digestion times. According to nutritionist and food-combining advocate Dr. Stanley Bass, water, juice, fruits and vegetables have generally short digestion times of under 45 minutes, and whole grains, dairy products, proteins, nuts, seeds and complex carbohydrates take more than one hour and sometimes as long as several hours to digest. Proponents of food combining believe that the stomach overworks when it digests a variety of foods at a single meal, and it's healthiest for the stomach to handle similar types of food at once. When the stomach has completed the majority of digestion for one group of items and is mostly empty, it's permissible to eat again.*

### *Good Combinations*

*Combine foods that have similar digestion times or that are in the same food group (with the exception of proteins, which should be limited to one type at each meal). Alder Brooke Healing Arts recommends combining vegetables with buttery or fatty foods, carbohydrates or proteins. Other good combinations include starches with carbohydrates or proteins and fatty foods with carbohydrates.*

### *Bad Combinations*

*Avoid combining starches and carbohydrates with proteins. Acidic foods and basic (alkaline) foods should be eaten separately as well. Fruits and most juices are composed largely of simple carbohydrates and take only a short time to digest; therefore, it's best to avoid consuming them with any other foods. Finally, desserts don't combine well with any meal. They are heavy in sugar, and food-combining advocates believe that they ferment in the stomach rather than digest easily.*

### Chewing

*People who follow the principles of food combining believe that it's important to completely chew all foods at all meals. Healing Daily also stresses the importance of chewing all foods thoroughly before swallowing them, almost to the point of liquidizing them. The organization notes that partially chewed food is almost always only partially digested and can pass through the body without fully dispersing its vitamins, minerals and nutrients."*

## Food combination vs. weight gain

The most common concern of almost every person is their weight as they age. They have tried almost all the diet plans around and yet most are still disappointed with the results. Some people offer weight loss programs at gyms and at yoga classes. However, not everyone have the luxury or time to do both.

So what makes food combining so promising when it comes to weight loss? Several studies have shown that increased intake of fruit, vegetables, dietary fibre, vitamins C and B6, beta-carotene and folate can help in reducing weight in a population of overweight adults and as supported by a study published in *Nutrition Research*. The rules are pretty simple and if followed will ensure the success of the much wanted shedding of unwanted weight.

Remember, fruits maybe nourishing and jam-packed with the vital vitamins and minerals but it is digested so quickly, so it doesn't mix well with starches and proteins. It's been said that yogurt is also very quick and easy to digest. Yogurt and all kinds of fruit go well together. Acidic fruits such as apples and oranges can be a particular problem if they are eaten too close to a starchy meal. Banana is the only really flexible fruit. It's quite starchy so banana is good with porridge and cereals but it is also easy to digest so goes well with yogurt. Eat fruit as a snack between meals or as a starter to a main course in other words, on an empty stomach. Or leave a gap between courses.

Some have tried doing the practice of food combining to lose weight by following the some simple rules.
- Eat starches and proteins apart
- Eat fruit separately
- Try and leave 15 to 30 minutes between main course and dessert
- Don't worry about food combining seven day every week, five is fine

There are still some who try to lose weight by losing their body fat. It is a fact that our body is seventy percent water. Little is known by many that having enough water in our body could help us lose weight. Water effectively flushes out the toxins that are in our body and thus a reduction in body fat. When one is bloated with excess water, it is said that drinking more water helps ease the bloat by helping to run the body more efficiently and thereby eventually lose that weight.

**Food combination for a youthful glow**

In article below by David Cowley, author of numerous articles in ant-aging, he shared his insights on food combining. It cannot be denied that the food combining of Dr. Hay has come a long way and many benefits could be attributed to it.

*"We all want to loose weight, look younger and feel healthier. Why not use the proper combinations of foods to accomplish this; after all we are what we eat. We may not be able to accomplish all of our goals but we can certainly slow down the effects of the aging process on our bodies. More and more people are discovering that combining the proper foods to reverse the aging process is a good start.*

*Food combination is the process of ingestion certain foods together while avoiding other food combinations altogether. This is not any type of diet where some foods are not eaten. It only means that certain combinations of foods are not eaten at the same time. The body takes different amount of time to digest different foods depending on the general type of food being eaten. For example, it is believed that you should not eat proteins with starchy foods or that acidic and alkaline foods should not to be eaten together.*

*If you go back far enough in human history you will conclude that eating different foods at the same time was not the norm. Humans wander around in small family groups looking for food. When then came upon a food source such as a nut for fruit tree or if they found or killed an animal it was eaten on the spot. If any of the food was left after the eating binge then the excess food may have been saved for later use.*

*The human body adapted to this food availability by producing different enzymes to digest different types of foods. Carbohydrates require carbohydrate digesting enzymes and Proteins require protein digesting enzymes. The production of protein enzymes and carbohydrate enzymes at the same time can lead can lead to indigestion, gas, cramping and the poor digestion of foods.*

*Here is a list of nine general rules for a proper food combination diet.*

*1) Carbohydrates (Bread, Potatoes, Rice, and Wheat) should not be eaten with Acidic Foods (Tomato, Pineapples, Grapefruits, and Oranges). Ptyalin enzyme is used to digest alkaline foods and is destroyed by acidic foods. The eating of acidic foods with carbohydrates can lead to a fermentation process that produces gas. Citrus fruits can safely be eaten as a snack from 30 minutes to 1 hour prior to a regular meal. Tomatoes can be eaten with green leafy vegetables and fatty foods.*

*2) Proteins (Meat, Cheese, Eggs, and Nuts) should not be eaten with Carbohydrates (Potatoes, Grains, Sweet Fruits, and most Desserts).*

*3) Two different Proteins at the same time. Do not combine Meat, Cheese, Eggs, Nuts, Milk. The enzyme require to digest proteins need to be in different strengths for different proteins.*

*4) Proteins and Fats. Eat only lean meats because fats will suppress the appetite thus retarding the production of protein digestive enzymes.*

*5) Proteins (Meat, Cheese, Eggs, and Nuts) should not be eaten with Acidic Foods (Tomato, Pineapples, Grapefruits, and Oranges). Same reasoning as rule 1.*

*6) Starches (Potatoes, Grains, and Cereals) should not be eaten with Sugars. Sugar causes the mouth to produce an excessive amount of saliva which will dilute the concentration of ptyalin in the stomach.*

*7) Starches (Potatoes, Grains, and Cereals) should not be eaten with other Starches.*

*8) Melons should always be eaten alone. The digestion of melons happens very quickly and can be eaten as a snack from 30 minutes to 1 hour prior to a regular meal.*

*9) Milk should always be ingested alone. Milk requires a very specific enzyme to be digested properly.*

*At first glance the above rules will not allow you to maintain a balance diet. You will still need to maintain a balance diet just do not eat a serving from each of the food groups at the same time. Divide up you eating day into smaller units with the correct combinations of foods in them will go a long way in your fight against the aging process. We need our bodies the chance to digest what we eat properly.*

*Proper food combining encourages you to eat healthily. You will be getting more of the vitamins and minerals your body needs. Your skin will become clearer and healthier looking. No more indigestion or gas, you will have more energy, no more limp hair or pasty skin. Food combining for anti-aging purposes is a great way to fight the rigors of time.*

*If you just feel that you need vitamins, supplements or herbs to fight the aging process then find a good health care professional prior to starting any type of home treatment."*

**Food combination to detoxify body**

Almost every human being wants to have a clean body, inside and out. With the pollution and all the dirt and toxins in the surroundings and in the food we eat, having a body detoxification frees us form the harmful radicals that affect our health and body.

So what is body detoxification all about? Body cleansing or detoxification is treatment in which the body gets rid of the accumulated harmful substances that have a negative effect on the individual's health.

Our body is not designed to eat and accumulate all kinds of food all at the same time, even with the healthy ones. Since our digestive enzymes have a requirement of a certain pH level in order to function. Proteins and some foods require longer time in the stomach as compared to other foods. Fats and oil coat our stomach lining making it more difficult for the stomach to secrete that much needed acid to digest food. When you decide to eat nuts and olive oil together, better think twice on your choice. Nuts are very hard to digest and olive oil makes it hard for the stomach to release the acid and digest the nuts.

So how does detoxification work? Basically, detoxification means cleaning the blood. It does this mainly by removing impurities from the blood in the liver, where toxins are processed for elimination. The body also eliminates toxins through the kidneys, intestines, lungs, lymph and skin. However, when this system is compromised, impurities aren't properly filtered and every cell in the body is adversely affected.

By combining foods properly, your digestion is well aided and the elimination of toxins in the body is achieved. We detoxify to be healthy and feel healthy. But being one isn't simply eating good food, it's about eating the good food in a right way at the right times. A good detox program can help the body's natural cleaning process by:

1) Resting the organs through fasting;
2) Stimulating the liver to drive toxins from the body;
3) Promoting elimination through the intestines, kidneys and skin;
4) Improving circulation of the blood; and
5) Refueling the body with healthy nutrients.

A detox program however must only be done once a year; perhaps a short one is enough and is good for your health. As a word of caution - All long-term fasts require medical supervision as well as prior assessment as to levels of nutrients, to ensure that deficiency does not occur. Weekend fasts are safe for most people, although it is still wise to seek advice from a professional experienced in detoxification

Some of the common detox methods include water and juice fast, weekend monodiet, alkaline-detoxification diet, Vitamin C therapy and Chelation therapy.

**Energetic with raw food combination**

When we overload our body with one huge meal, this has a detrimental effect to our over-all energy level. All the energy we have is being directed to the digestive system in order to properly digest what we have just eaten. An overload on eating will never do any good but it will even make us sleepy and tired.

So what could be the foods that would boost up our energy level? I for one firmly believe that raw food could significantly improve our energy level as well as our performance. Performance is meant to be our daily activity and how we are doing and feeling every minute of it.

Caffeine and sugar in our beverages and food is one good energy booster bit only for a certain if not brief time. When its effect wears out, we too feel worn out. We feel drained and have to get another energy boost.

Raw foods are very easy to digest as they have these enzymes to aid our body in digestion and other processes. Raw foods are in the original state making them very digestible and so the body will no longer waste any additional energy to digest them. Aside from easy to digest, raw foods are jam packed with nutrients as compared to cooked food. Compared to junk foods which contain empty calories and less Nutritional value, raw foods are the best snack to have.

Most people will notice that they will get more energy when juicing vegetables like carrots and celery. Any kind of vegetables is sure to have those energy boosters and what could be better than drinking natural fruits and vegetable juice.

So, what do you eat on a raw food diet? A raw food diet is given by one who has doing it for years.

- **Salads.** Lots of fresh, green, organic vegetables. And the more variety, the better. And the ideal dressing is cold-pressed extra virgin olive oil with herbs, spices and orange or lemon juice. But, you could get away with the olive oil and balsamic vinegar.
- **Juices.** It's best to get a good quality juicer. Try not to buy the bottled juices from the store. Juicing at home will allow you to take in "fresh" juices with all the minerals, vitamins and enzymes that your body needs.
- **Nuts and Seeds.** Raw, organic nuts and seeds, eaten within moderation (and sprinkled into salads) will give the body much needed protein, good fats and calories for energy. Go easy on the nuts and seeds. Use sparingly, and mix them into other foods like salads and raw vegan sushi.

- **Fruits.** If you're not juicing them, eat them! Raw, organic fresh fruits are an excellent source of nutrition and energy. Apples and oranges. Still common but essential fruits to eat daily to boost one's energy level. Also, bananas are great as well. And grapes as well as all the berries (especially blueberries) contain antioxidants to help fight against cancer.
- **Aloe Vera.** This is somewhat of a miracle plant that many researchers are still puzzled about regarding its beneficial properties. Aloe Vera juice provides many benefits, like healing and rejuvenation of the body's cells. In fact, many people around the world will cut a leaf from the Aloe Vera plant and use the juice to apply to a cut or burn to make it heal faster. Taken as a juice, Aloe Vera helps heal the body and give it more energy, and at the same time aiding in digestion and allowing more nutrients to be absorbed. Always buy the raw, organic Aloe Vera juice for best results.

## Conclusion

To recap, the food combining system, as a whole, is simple and easy to understand. It logically evolved from the study of gastric physiology and the actions of enzymes and digestive juices. It is not what we eat, but what we digest and assimilate, that determines the nourishment our bodies receive. Food combining is based on the discovery that certain combinations of food may be digested with greater ease and efficiency than others.

Food combining improves our overall health and outlook. But this could only be achieved if the diet is done properly and religiously. When the combinations are done as told or instructed, we will feel fresh, energetic, young and light.

But the method could only do so much. It still depends on us on how we do things and how we look at it. We cannot expect to result after a day. A program whose results could be seen almost immediately is not good news. Good results come from time and the determination of the one doing it.

What is important is that at the end of the day, you feel satisfied and contented!